Narrating the New Predictive Genetics

This book explores the way changes in technology have altered the relationship between ethics and medicine. For some inherited diseases, new genetic testing technologies may provide much more accurate diagnostic and predictive information which raises important questions about consent, confidentiality and the use of information by family members and other third parties. What are the implications of this knowledge for individuals and their families? And for society more widely? How should this new information be used? How do people deal with the apparent choices that new knowledge and technologies offer? Drawing on extensive ethnographic research with families affected by Huntington's Disease and using perspectives from medical and cultural anthropology, the author explores the huge disparity between the experience of living with the results of genetic testing and the knowledge and expertise which are drawn on to develop policy and clinical services.

MONICA KONRAD teaches at the Department of Social Anthropology, University of Cambridge and directs the PLACEB-O research group (Partners Linked Across Collaborations in Ethics and the Biosciences – Orbital). Her research addresses the relevance of contemporary anthropology for global governance in science, international ethics and interdisciplinary studies. She is the author of *Nameless Relations: Anonymity, Melanesia and Reproductive Gift Exchange between British Ova Donors and Recipients* and currently acts as anthropological advisor to bioethics councils in the UK and for the UN.

Cambridge Studies in Society and the Life Sciences

Series Editors
Nikolas Rose, *London School of Economics*
Paul Rabinow, *University of California at Berkeley*

This interdisciplinary series focuses on the social shaping, social meaning and social implications of recent developments in the life sciences, biomedicine and biotechnology. It places original research and innovative theoretical work within a global, multi-cultural context.

Other titles in series

Narrating the New Predictive Genetics

Ethics, Ethnography and Science

MONICA KONRAD
University of Cambridge

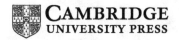

CAMBRIDGE
UNIVERSITY PRESS

CAMBRIDGE
UNIVERSITY PRESS

University Printing House, Cambridge CB2 8BS, United Kingdom

One Liberty Plaza, 20th Floor, New York, NY 10006, USA

477 Williamstown Road, Port Melbourne, VIC 3207, Australia

314-321, 3rd Floor, Plot 3, Splendor Forum, Jasola District Centre, New Delhi - 110025, India

103 Penang Road, #05-06/07, Visioncrest Commercial, Singapore 238467

Cambridge University Press is part of the University of Cambridge.

It furthers the University's mission by disseminating knowledge in the pursuit of education, learning and research at the highest international levels of excellence.

www.cambridge.org
Information on this title: www.cambridge.org/9780521540667

First published 2005

A catalogue record for this publication is available from the British Library

ISBN 978-0-521-54066-7 Paperback

For my mother

Contents

III   RELATIONAL ETHICS IN PRACTICE

Acknowledgements

This project had its genesis in an Economic and Social Research Council funded research study I began in 1997–98 ('Culture, Kinship and Ethics in the Context of the New Reproductive and Genetic Technologies' [R000222290]). Over the years numerous organisations have made this research possible and numerous others have facilitated its progression. I thank first all the families who agreed to take part in the research and welcomed me into their lives, often in trying circumstances. Most of all to everyone who insisted on sharing their insights and made the research 'theirs', so to speak. The members of the HDA (Huntington's Disease Association) Dorset Branch were good enough to invite me to their support group activities and committee meetings. I must thank Hedley Thomas for his warm hospitality during my visits. Thanks also to Trudi Smith and the HDA South Hampshire Branch for their invitations to present work-in-progress. Sue Watkin and Cath Stanley of the HDA helped with such enthusiasm and kindness at the early stages of the research, putting me in touch with many of their friends and colleagues, and I was fortunate to be able to consult with Wendy Watson of the Hereditary Breast Cancer National Helpline who opened my eyes to other realities. For their assiduous attention to detail, I thank all the assistants who helped to transcribe the lengthy transcripts of taped interviews.

Mention too must be made of the dedicated campaign work of Human Genetics Alert, the Genetics Interest Group and GeneWatch UK whose staff have helped to keep me on track. Learning also about the strategy of 'horizon scoping' has provided another welcome entry route into the world of predictive science. The openness of the Human Genetics Commission (HGC), an advisory body reporting to the UK government, to expose its working methods and the willingness of Commissioners to debate before the public at its open plenary meetings gives fresh hope to the immanence of ethical accountability within all committee life. I thank Baroness Helena Kennedy, QC, Chair of the HGC and Professor Alexander McCall Smith, Vice-Chair, for setting the example.

Additional thanks to the HGC Secretariat for help with research enquiries along the way.

For letting me shadow them periodically in 1998 during their clinical interactions with patients, I extend my appreciation to Professor Kay McDermott and nurse genetic counsellor Wendy Chorley at the Royal Free Hospital, London. Chris Mathew and Liz Green, Division of Medical and Molecular Genetics, Guy's Hospital, London and Alison Lashwood, Guy's Hospital, also showed and explained the more technical side of things inside laboratory space. Professors Peter Harper, University of Wales College of Medicine in Cardiff and Bernadette Modell, University College London Medical School, Gerrit Dommerholt of International Huntington's Association, Dr Nancy Wexler, Columbia University, New York and Prof Ira Shoulson, University of Rochester, were kind enough to respond to points of concern and generously forwarded relevant publications. And in the 'in-between' spaces where science and ethics properly intersect, the intellectual inspiration of colleagues from the International Council for Science, especially their commitment to the future of international, cross-cultural and multi-disciplinary endeavours, has helped again to keep me on track.

Small parts of Chapters 3 and 4 were used to a different purpose in my journal articles, 'Predictive genetic testing and the making of the pre-symptomatic person: prognostic moralities amongst Huntington's affected families', *Anthropology and Medicine*, 10(1):23–49 (2003); and 'From secrets of life to the life of secrets: tracing genetic knowledge as genealogical ethics in biomedical Britain', *The Journal of the Royal Anthropological Institute*, 9(2):339–58 (2003). I am grateful to the Royal Anthropological Institute of Great Britain and Ireland and the editors and publishers of this material for permission to use it here. My thanks to Martin Rowson for permission to reproduce his wonderful cartoon in the Introduction.

Monica Konrad
London
December 2003

Introduction

Predictive genetic testing technology is still very much in its infancy in Western healthcare systems. However, as geneticists continue to establish links between the location of genes and particular disease aetiology, so further scientific knowledge may occasion more encompassing social definitions of who legitimately can be classified as 'pre-ill' or 'pre-symptomatic'. Potentially all of us may be transformed into 'genetic citizens' with one kind or another of genetic 'profile', either before birth or sometime during our life course. But what exactly does it mean to be classified as a person with a predisposition to illness and how are the life sciences and technologies creating pre-symptomatic persons as new forms of social value?

This book is a critical exploration of the emerging pre-emptive cultures that shape the new predictive genetics. Based on original materials from fieldwork in contemporary Britain, it argues there is a pressing need for the social sciences to analyse conceptually, empirically and pragmatically how we think through the links that bind together the ideals of prophecy and health in such predictive contexts.

The ethical controversies surrounding genetic testing have largely emerged since the development of tests based on the direct analysis of a person's DNA. This has only been possible since the identification of bio-molecular markers enabled geneticists to begin the work of tracing correlations between particular disease-causing agents and specific genes. Though successful linkage applies still mainly to the 'single-gene' disorders whose genetic mutations are considerably simpler to study than the more common polygenic conditions, scientific understanding of the nature of multiple interactions between different sets of genes in disease formation is commonly heralded as the next genetics 'revolution'. The possibility for genetic diagnosis itself, though, is not entirely new. Antenatal testing for chromosomal abnormalities such as Down's syndrome has been offered routinely to older pregnant women and genetic screening already has some routine applications. In the UK, all newborn babies are screened for phenylketonuria, a genetic condition that can lead to serious learning difficulties unless counteracted by a special diet. For babies that test positively, the adverse effects can be pre-empted by early treatment.

It is this kind of example about the merits of early illness prevention and treatment that underpins rationalisations for the promise of a 'golden age' of new predictive healthcare. These rationalisations are underwritten by many of the late-capitalist economies of the West that aim to link advances in future health provision with supremacist ideas of cultural progress and power. The biosciences and life technologies are endowed in many of these visions with an implicit civilising mission. Britain, for example, aspires 'to lead the world in the discovery and realisation of the maximum benefits of genetics in healthcare', with the British government pledged to invest £50 million in genetic research, genetics-based health services and professional training between 2003–6, with further funding to follow (Department of Health 2003:8). Elevating in this way the gene to the newly enhanced status of visible cultural icon, it is only by appreciating the wider social implications of the predictive testing era that the claims of the original guiding promise will be open to critical scrutiny and ongoing evaluation (see figure page 3).

Taking a strong integrative approach that draws out some of the possibilities for a productive synthesis between social anthropology, cultural analysis and a critical bioethics, *Narrating the New Predictive Genetics* introduces a number of important empirical findings that extend the parameters of existing critiques of 'geneticisation' in significant new directions. The aim here is to contribute to a growing social science scholarship on the anthropology, sociology and psychology of the new genetics (e.g., Rabinow 1999; Conrad and Gabe 1999; Marteau and Richards 1996) by paying attention to how we formulate questions about the meaning of predictive genetic knowledge for definitions of society. Both the anthropology of biomedicine and the cultural analysis of new genetic technologies are relatively recent topics within the social sciences. A few anthropologists, for instance, have turned their attention to women's experiences of prenatal screening techniques as well as interpretations of risk amongst those undertaking predispositional screening for breast cancer (Rapp 1999; Finkler 2000; Lock 1998; for other monographs addressing the new genetics see Rabinow 1996, 1999; Fujimura 1996; see also Franklin and Lock 2003). However there has been no critical study devoted to the shift from treatment to prevention-based medicines, and in particular no anthropological study exploring how the making of the 'pre-symptomatic person' reconfigures current definitions of sociality and social identity in complex, technologically

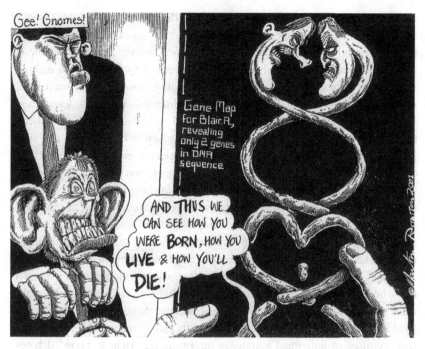

Gee! Gnomes!
"And **thus** we can see how you were **born**, how you **live** and how you'll **die!**"
12 February 2001
Reproduced by kind permission of *The Guardian*. © Martin Rowson 2001.

This political cartoon uses the 'breakthrough' of the first so-called 'rough draft'
of the sequenced human genome to illustrate the potentially determinist reasoning
behind predictive claims to genetic supremacy. In this case, a satirical play on
the nature of political power depicts the internal rivalry between two government
figures from the current Labour Party in Britain: the Chancellor of the Exchequer,
Mr Gordon Brown, is shown finally to supersede the Prime Minister, Mr Tony Blair
whose genome comically reveals next to no genes.

advanced societies. This is a somewhat strange omission, for ever since E. E.
Evans-Pritchard's (1937) seminal *Witchcraft, Oracles, and Magic among the*
Azande, social anthropologists have attended to the many ways that divinatory
knowledge across non-Western cultures is believed to have transformative effect
through the medium of manipulated human bodies and other ritualised objects.
Revisiting then something of an 'old' anthropological interest, this book offers a
critical commentary on the new oracular predispositional 'truths' of twenty-first
century prophetic biology and the relation of these truths to changing popular
conceptions of persons, bodies and notions of genetic inheritance in biomedical
Britain today.

By way of detailed case studies of families affected by Huntington's Disease (HD) – a monogenic (single-gene) inherited and late-onset condition for which there is presently no known cure – we will examine how the exchange of genetic information between kin entails unresolved processes of moral decision-making within and across the generations. Understanding, however, why such local moralities of information disclosure generate dilemmas over what knowledge is 'good' to know and what knowledge is 'bad' to tell and share with others, raises questions of wide relevance beyond the specifics of HD cases and sub-jective illness experiences. To date, anthropologically informed commentaries of the new medical technologies have largely neglected the conceptual ques-tion of how, and to what extent, the choices informing people's reproductive and genetic decision-making comprise so-called 'ethnographies of morality' (Howell 1997). As a consequence, anthropologists interested in this area have tended to avoid asking how, and indeed how adequately, their conceptual appa-ratus can address the working premises of mainstream Western bioethics. In the context of predictive genetic testing technology where consanguineal ('blood') kin who have chosen not to get tested may find another's test result impli-cates their own health status, such issues become especially germane. In the light of these difficult disclosure dilemmas, this study reconsiders the concep-tual premises of individual autonomy informing the 'right to know' debates of contemporary Western bioethics. It finds the interrelatedness of interests informing local practices particularly suggestive for the conceptualisation of a 'genealogical ethics', which in turn may be seen as part of a wider relational amalgam (a 'relational ethics'). Additionally, I have wanted to introduce certain cross-cultural data from the existing medical anthropological record to show why such materials are salient to the wider discussion of human embodiment and identity in the genome era. Since the inclusion of comparative data has been noticeably absent from previous ethnographies of the new medical tech-nologies, such comparisons hopefully yield additional interest and broaden the terms of debate, for anthropologists and non-anthropologists alike.

In the course of researching this book, I have lost track of the number of times people have asked questions about my intellectual allegiances. For whom does one write? To whom is one talking? For all authors, these are impor-tant, inescapable questions. As indicated, the following pages are attuned to particular anthropological sensibilities, however I want to stress that the book is written at the same time with a broader non-anthropological readership in mind. Indeed one main aim is to bring together the usually disparate domains of ethics, ethnography and science as the beginning of a critical exploration in interdisciplinary dialogue between medical and non-medical practitioners. During their daily rounds, clinical geneticists, genetic counsellors and academic bioethicists usually do not 'talk with' social scientists. Just the same might be said of the latter: social scientists rarely find themselves positioned as well-integrated or long-term fixtures within mainstream scientific or medical research communities. Issues of access to clinical settings by non-clinicians are often the first impediment to such cross-dialogue. But these disciplinary and inter-institutional 'gaps' between the different practices and scholarly communities seem, if anything, more essential to address now as shifts towards so-called 'Mode-2' distributed knowledge production demand new transparency and participatory structures.

When an ethnographer chooses to work with and through certain publics – when he or she purposely mediates the creative space of the 'agora' (Nowotny *et al.* 2002) – then engaging the professional interest of scientists, clinical geneticists and other health professionals seriously matters. Let me be specific. Since the rate of uptake of predictive genetic testing has been far lower amongst the HD community than was originally expected by clinicians, there is a dearth of social knowledge relating to the real life experiences of genetically predisposed (i.e., 'at risk') but untested individuals. There is also very little public awareness of what it means for affected families and individuals to live with a 'pre-symptomatic' diagnosis. Living life pre-symptomatically is a skill few us might have heard about at the present time. Indeed, clinicians themselves have cited evidence suggesting that those who experience the greatest difficulty in coping with an adverse test result are also the likeliest client group to drop out of clinical follow-up studies. Similarly, although policy specialists often pay lip service to the 'ethical dilemmas' of predictive genetic testing technology, the normative formulation of bioethical statements on predictive testing by various expert committees has been delimited extremely narrowly. Across Euro-America, relevant ethical bodies have not to date focused on broad inclusive questions such as how revised diagnostic tools in clinical genetics are creating 'pre-symptomatic' persons as new social identities. In the media too, there has been next to no debate addressing how the effects of these genetic testing technologies are creating new prognostic moralities of 'foreknowledge' at the level of ordinary lived experience. Based on the 'expert' accounts of those who have tested positively as well as those receiving good news, this book by contrast reorients the focus through illustrative examples and stories from specific contexts. With its close attention to narrativisation and issues of temporality it hopes to supplement the quantitative research which clinicians routinely consult and analyse.

PART I

Ethnography as linkage map

1
Thinking futures

Lives to come

In 1994 the late French novelist and literary translator Elizabeth Gille published a remarkable autobiography about temporal dating and anticipated death. Realising her diagnosis of terminal cancer leaves limited creative writing time, Gille pens *Le Crabe sur la Banquette Arrière*, the story of a counterpart heroine who tries to put her remaining days of declining health to the back of her mind. Friends, colleagues, family and even strangers all have other plans, however. Meaning well, they rally round this 'sick' relation offering clippings from popular magazines on the latest 'miracle remedies'; or they collect groceries suggesting she eat a 'healthy' fish diet, cook these recipes, do those exercises and so on. To her frustration Gille's heroine is reminded continuously by others how her designated sickness role, as enforced regimen of care, predates her impending death. As the author herself remarked in the advanced stages of her illness, these kinship relations are however misplaced conceptions. 'The date of your deaths remains uncertain, but mine is already set, more or less', she told close friends. 'That does not prevent me from living. Or from laughing'.[1]

It is no accident that the recent ascendancy of new genetic testing technologies primarily in the wealthiest markets of the late industrialised world has spawned both a sceptical and optimistic literature about the 'dream' of the human genome and of future 'lives to come' (see Lewontin 2000; Kitcher 1996). Scientists, the media, industry, bio-pharmaceutical companies each have various 'stories' to tell and venture interests to perpetrate about the intended benefits derived from the future creation of supposedly healthier populations. In its extreme version the vision anticipates a new era of cheap rapid genetic screening with technologies such as the DNA chip and personalised sequencing. Go to your primary care practitioner and theoretically he or she will be able to predict the probability of your getting any number of known genetic diseases, including the common multi-factorial conditions such as heart disease, cancer and diabetes. On this basis, one's doctor could hope to recommend preventive measures before certain symptoms appear. You might be advised to come for regular check-ups, modify your diet, quit smoking, take more exercise, avoid environmental toxins and so on. Alternatively, the genetic consumer might bypass altogether the medical specialist and simply go to the local pharmacy instead. Just as 'do-it-yourself' DNA testing kits are appearing already on the market today – sold 'over-the-counter', available via the Internet or through alternative practitioners (e.g. dieticians, complementary therapists) – so in the future one might purchase one's own DNA sequence directly as a disk to self-analyse at home on one's personal computer.[2]

But would we all live longer, healthier and happier lives as a result? For the major pharmaceutical and biotechnology companies, the question may be tangential to other prime considerations. Namely, the perceived benefits of pre-dispositional profiling turn in part on the generation of near-term revenue and the return of pharmaceutical profit for previously patented genes. The expansion of the drug market to 'pills for the healthy ill' may also precipitate onerous forms of commercial and psychological exploitation through the manipulative 'marketing of fear'; something of an antidote to the calculations of pharmacogenetics and pre-emptively tailored individual drug responses (Gilham and Rowland 2001; Moynihan *et al.* 2002; see also Davison *et al.* 1994). Such concerns tend to be countered in existing policy debate by the presumption of the active information-seeking subject and the belief that expected benefits for the populace at large turn on the individual's supposedly free choice to make responsible genetic interventions to stave off disease – this especially so against an ideological backdrop of advanced liberalism and active citizenship (for sociological critiques see Novas and Rose 2000; Koch 1999). Across these concerns one hears some research geneticists articulating the intellectual caution brake. Apparently doubtful of the predictive power of genetic medicine for the treatment of polygenic complex disorders, such developments – it is claimed – are at least some twenty to thirty years away. Of course such doubt may serve at times as another promotional strategy: the scientists' assuagement of the public's confidence. A recent refrain at academic conferences and 'science and society' events goes along the lines: 'Don't worry – things aren't running out of control – the complexity of risk quantification for common disorders is way beyond [even] us!' Meanwhile, the goal of developing a radical breakthrough (in terms of cost and throughput) in sequencing of genomic DNA has been captured in the slogan 'the thousand dollar genome' (i.e. sequencing the whole genome of an individual for about $1k in about a day). This was first articulated at a 'visionary meeting' organised by the National Human Genome Research Institute (NHGRI) and chaired by Francis Collins in 2002.[3] In conveying these various rationalisations to the public, certain sectors of the media tend to muddle and simplify the picture with inaccurate reportage of scientists finding genes 'for' certain conditions, as if genomic-based science were fundamentally a matter of straightforward causal correlation between a gene and the phenotype, to say nothing of differences in social structure, lifestyle and environment. Through these overlapping and oft contradictory claims 'Biotechnology' mixes benefits with harms in one seamless package such that the knowledge outcomes of the Human Genome Project often collide in a supercharged vacuum of gung-ho determinist triumphacy. A collision that anthropologist Paul Rabinow (1999:23) derides as the 'hyperbolic discursive tidal wave of hope, fear and metadiscourse', and one that some clinically trained practitioners condemn with equal opprobrium as the dangers of a new age of medicalisation and rhetorical hype (Holtzman and Marteau 2000; see also Melzer and Zimmern 2002).

It is precisely such sensationalism strategies that I want to move away from so as to reorient debate through a different analytic trajectory. By traversing the conventionally discrete domains of ethics and science in post-Enlightenment European philosophy, this book unfolds as a cultural exploration of the way ethnographic analysis can be deployed as a critical tool to mediate the worlds of objective scientific 'fact' and subjective ethical 'value'. Part 1, 'Ethnography as linkage map', outlines some key themes and locates the nature of the ethnographic problem in terms of a culturally resonant 'linkage map'. Before I start to sketch in these points of linkage, let me account a little more explicitly for some of the ethnographer's own concerns. Social scientists may be trained to deride hype, but such critical detachment does not abstain me from participatory engagement, albeit more subtle and reflexive forms of involvement. Nobody after all can write as though they were *tabula rasa*.

I want to present three caveats along the way. The first is nothing more than an acknowledgement. It is to make the rather simple but critical point that a wide range of genetic tests with different degrees of predictability is currently under development. It is then seriously misleading to talk about predictive medicine as though it were a monolithic enterprise, since in so doing we underplay the significant difference between those high-risk families with a known hereditary illness (single-gene inherited diseases) and common complex diseases in the wider population (Mathew 2001). For the latter, the presence of gene variations or 'polymorphisms' may mean that genes represent fairly poor predictors of disease. Take the example of workplace hazards and the case of an employer wishing to test job applicants with a predictive susceptibility test prior to the offer of an employment contract. Now a person's potential susceptibility to a chemical could be affected by hundreds of different genes that encode enzymes and molecules involved in many different metabolic pathways. Rather than any single genetic difference it may be the overall pattern of gene variation that will influence the possible onset of a health problem. Or genetic differences may be attributable to different metabolic transfer rates whose effects cannot be easily predicted. You may be able to break down toxic chemicals efficiently that prevent the development of a predispositional risk factor, whereas my body might not produce the right level of enzymes in the right amount, even though I feel and appear quite healthy. If we both keep our distance from the group of chemicals known as arylamines (associated with dyes, textiles and rubber manufacture), then theoretically our different metabolic rates as fast and slow 'acetylators' will be of negligible predictive value for the NAT2 gene variation linked with the increased susceptibility risk to bladder cancer. But the added caveat reveals the complex subtleties at work. The genetic variation in NAT2 that is thought to increase the risk of bladder cancer is also thought to reduce the risk of developing colon cancer. All in all, I may be more protected from colon disease than you! Any predictive genetic test result could therefore involve the misinterpretation of an individual's actual risk, thereby leading to social inequality through practices of genetic discrimination – my not getting the job appointment, for example.[4]

Second, as more tests for multi-factorial genetic disorders become available in the coming years in the form of so-called 'pre-dispositional' diagnostics, we need to think much more carefully about what is meant by the umbrella term 'preventive health'. This is especially so since preventive genetic medicine is couched so often in terms of helpful treatments and effective care, omitting to say that health prevention as a practice and ideology is also tied up closely with the political economy of health systems. If health policy administrators keep an interested eye on developments in the new life technologies, this is partly because it will be more cost effective to 'screen out' persons preconceptively or to treat certain conditions prophylactically, than it will be to subsidise the cost of long-term care for those with chronic symptoms. The National Institute for Clinical Excellence (NICE) produces for the National Health Service in England and Wales authoritative guidance on the clinical and cost effective-ness of healthcare interventions and on the treatment of clinical conditions. NICE has already produced clinical guidelines in familial breast cancer and undertaken appraisals for two medicinal products, trastuzumab (Herceptin) and imatinib (Glivec) that require the prior genetic analysis of tumour cells before they are prescribed (Department of Health 2003:52). Sociological critiques of 'surveillance medicine' and 'genetic governmentality' have addressed already such important issues as medicines access within the larger cultural framework of social justice (see e.g. Armstrong 1995; Rose 1990; Kerr 2003). These critiques rightly stress the need to challenge and negotiate discursive claims that implicitly or explicitly seek to justify certain links between predictive medicine and new encroaching forms of bio-surveillance, for instance in the testing and selection of persons in employment, education and insurance contexts.

Third, predictive genetic testing also raises new questions and dilemmas for families. A common feature of genetic tests for diseases of Mendelian pattern of inheritance concerns the fact that an individual's test result usually has implications for other family members. Genetics affects more than ego; it is profoundly relational since one's genetic inheritance may bind the self to others. Genes do not just provide an individual with identity, they also 'relate persons to one another and give them an identity as 'relatives' (Strathern 1995:104). When knowledge about a person's anticipated health can become systematised as new predictive genetic information that is not only relevant to the testee but also to all his or her consanguineal kin, what exactly does it mean to talk of genetic futures? As the sociologists Alan Petersen and Robin Bunton observe, the new genetics as applied to public health will profoundly transform our concepts of self as embodied beings. 'It is in its potential to alter our view of ourselves and of our relationships with others that the new genetics has its most potent effects as a form of governance' (Petersen and Bunton 2002:30). What then happens to the link between culture and health when people start to anticipate social relations primarily as the time between diagnosis and an embodied prognosis, and when – perhaps most importantly of all – the remedy of a potential cure is still pending? Can everybody just continue to *laugh* like Elizabeth Gille in the face of changing conceptions of genetic heredity? And how are these new life technologies of prediction reconfiguring our understandings of moral obligation as modern familial forms of 'kinship ethics'?

In *The Voice of Prophecy*, anthropologist Edwin Ardener (1989) identified some of the pervasively elusive and paradoxical features inherent in both the idea and temporality of prophecy. Before they happen, prophetic situations may seem strange events without any comprehensible meaning or wider socio-cultural validation. In retrospect, however, the enduring effects of these situations often may seem so mundane and trivial that their instancing as new ideational associations seems barely recognisable as particular cultural forces *already* underway. Ardener's important theoretical point, developed as the 'prophetic condition', stressed that those claiming prophetic foresight do not in fact predict the future in terms of the present. Rather, they foretell a present situation before it has been culturally validated and naturalised through linguistic representation. The prophetic condition, therefore, if it is to have any cultural salience, manifests itself as a new discursive language and puts into articulation the cultural contours of another social reality.

In examining various aspects of predictive medicine as a new discursive language, this book asks how contemporary developments in genetic science are shaping the contours of prophetic reality. To such ends, our enquiry probes extensively the emerging armoury of pre-symptomatic classification. Whereas diagnostic genetic testing is seen as appropriate for individuals already displaying particular symptoms, and more or less verifies or further refines diagnostic judgement about the presence of a particular disease, pre-symptomatic genetic testing is carried out on persons medically categorised and subsequently 'revealed' (or precluded from social labelling) as 'pre-symptomatic'.[5] As an extended commentary on the classificatory and ethical systems that support genetic governmentality through the creation of 'pre-symptomatic' value, *Narrating the New Predictive Genetics* pays close analytic and ethnographic attention to the lived condition that is the making of the pre-symptomatic person. We will hear the detailed testimonies from subjects who have undergone predictive genetic testing for a particular adult-onset monogenic (single-gene) condition. Others similarly share their real-life thoughts and anticipations enabling 'contexts to speak back' as the production of socially robust knowledge (Nowotny, Scott and Gibbons 2002). There are those who remain undecided as to whether they should get themselves tested pre-emptively 'ahead of illness' and spouses who find out they have married into an affected family once they have already had children. These are just some of the non-professional 'expert' voices detailing what gets spoken and what otherwise gets left unsaid in the co-evolving biocultures of prophetic genetics and society.

Hearing such voices from the ground is important for many reasons. For one thing, such articulations dovetail or cut across contemporary public policy debates over the uses of sensitive genetic information. Identifying a potential population of pre-symptomatic persons enables, of course, the collection of pre-emptively classifiable information about subjects' future health and well being. Such 'pre-emptive' capacities raise in turn many ethical and practical issues about data protection and the very notion of 'genetic privacy'. In Britain the ends to which genetic information can be put, particularly in the case of the establishment of human genetic databases and related issues of confidentiality and anonymisation, has been identified as an ethical and legal problem beyond the remit of scientific innovation and medical practice alone (House of Lords 2001). In its discussion document 'Whose Hands on Your Genes', the Human Genetics Commission (2000) notes several reasons why personal genetic information may be seen as special and treated differently from other medical information.

(1) It is unique to each person (except for 'identical' twins).
(2) It is technically possible to obtain it from a very small bodily sample without a person's consent.
(3) It can be used to predict disorders a person may develop in the future and may tell other family relatives about disorders they may develop too.
(4) These predictions can be of interest to others such as insurance companies or employers.
(5) It has a potential commercial value to organisations introducing developments based on genetic information.

As we shall see, the question of whether genetic information needs to be protected in a different way to other personal medical information is clearly a public health concern of interest to everyone, and not just health advisors and practitioners. The claim of 'genetic exceptionalism' is made all the more explicit a social problem in the context of an encroaching 'consumer genetics' and the commercialisation of 'do-it-yourself' self-testing home kits for certain conditions or susceptibilities. As the technology of predictive genetic testing moves gradually beyond the specialised field and expertise of the medical genetics clinic, so the issue of the status of genetic information begs the increasingly pervasive cultural question: how does pre-emptive genetic knowledge make out of persons moral systems of foreknowledge?

Bodies into oracles

The entry of the 'anthropologist as diviner' in such prophetic contexts is never a straightforward or isolated act. S/he experiments first in the consultative exercise of anticipatory ethnography in order to foretell certain pre-emptive futures and in this sense comes to be directly implicated in the engagement of ethical process and deliberation. As we shall see, the event of foretelling takes place partly through the literal work of a narrative ethics that challenges sociobiological conceptions of an evolutionary ethics (see Chapter 2 'Sociobiology as a new modern synthesis?'). In the ethnographic chapters (Parts II–III) we witness this as the workings of a locally conceived 'kinship ethics' put into practice as a temporally inflected 'genealogical ethics'. But the narrative ethics of foretelling and the ongoing kinship work of disclosure happen also to entail asking related questions about the responsibilities of 'applied anthropology' and issues of research advocacy. How, for instance, can we ensure that the ability to perform pre-symptomatic tests will not be transposed at some future moment into the normative imperative to have oneself genetically tested? If such conjecture seems far-fetched and if memories of past eugenicist abuse are thought sufficient a political check, then just listen to the plea for a 'psychocivilised society' advanced as recently as the late 1960s by Linus Pauling. A respected Nobel Prize winner on two occasions, once for chemistry and once for peace, Pauling was to advocate:

> there should be tattooed on the forehead of every young person a symbol showing possession of the sickle-cell gene or whatever other similar gene . . . It is my opinion that legislation along this line, compulsory testing for defective genes before marriage, and some form of public or semi-public display of this possession, should be adopted.
>
> *(Quotation from Linus Pauling [1968:269] cited in Kay [1993:276])*

At the present time there are growing public concerns about the potential eugenic aspects of emergent genetic knowledge. Many are inclined to see certain analogies between current developments in the 'new genetics' and former state-sanctioned eugenic practices prevalent in parts of Europe and North America. Others disagree that any meaningful comparisons can be made between the old style coercive eugenics and the so-called 'new eugenics' (see e.g., Kerr and Shakespeare 2002; Petersen and Bunton 2002:35–66; Hubbard and Wald 1993: 23–38; Rifkin 1998:128–29; Proctor 1992). In the light of such claims it is worth bearing in mind that whilst developing his thesis on the 'birth of the clinic' in Western biomedicine, Michel Foucault would often speak of Georges Canguilhelm, his theoretical mentor, as a 'philosopher of error' (Foucault 1966: xix). Canguilhelm, for his part, had argued against a view of pathology as homologous with the intrinsic physiology of a specific biological (and cultural) organism. Whatever is classified as 'abnormal', he insisted, could only be evaluated in terms of relationships. 'Life is what is capable of error . . . [and] . . . the concept of error, like the concept of pathology, is polysemic' (Foucault *ibid*, paraphrasing Canguilhelm). Of course it is almost something of a truism to say today that new biotechnological applications have opened an arena for contests of power over what it means to be human, as well as how and who has the power to define what counts as 'normal'. As ever, hype and sensationalism galvanise public interest, in part, through certain media representations. And no less so amongst scientific communities keen to attract large research funding grants. Criminologists, psychologists, social welfare workers, family therapists and others may also see a direct application here to genetics behavioural-ism debates (Nuffield Council on Bioethics 2002). But people do not become magically more or less 'normal' or 'human' *because* molecular biologists have identified the corporeal location of particular genes, and can hope to understand better the partial implication of these biochemical structures in human disease aetiology and illness incidence. Nor can cultural organisms appear to 'disappear' any the more effectively simply because these same scientists can point to the similarity of deoxyribonucleic acid content between (say) a human, chimpanzee or banana. As social science critiques of 'genetic fetishism' and 'geneticisation' have stressed so well (e.g. Lippman 1993; Rose 1997; Rapp 1999; Finkler 2000), these scientific developments have to be translated to particular contexts and particular persons in order for their cultural and ethical salience to carry any kind of socially meaningful 'predictive' value. Nonetheless Pauling's comments and similar utterances cannot be overlooked. They serve as a wake-up call for the ease with which future scenarios can already be introduced into public consciousness in terms of what presently seem palatable 'get out' clauses (cf. Ardener's [1989] 'prophetic condition'; cf. Duster's [1990] 'backdoor'). Once genetic testing technology is routinised as mass screening programmes and broadly institutionalised as part of what in the late 1980s was already identified as 'the new diagnostics' (Nelkin and Tancredi 1989:3–19), how will an adult's future personal decision *not* to take a genetic (predisposition) test be respected as a legitimate and 'normal' choice?[6] How do we imagine to ourselves the need to ensure such 'choice' is not represented by medical elites and biotechnological venture capital as a moral failure of courage, or else reduced simply to the personal whim to 'remain ignorant' of important 'revelatory' (read: cost efficient) knowledge? As the UK's Human Genetics Commission (2000:19) notes in the context of contemporary debates about the 'right to know' and 'not to know' genetic information, to what extent should we – and can we – protect people from unwanted knowledge about their genetic status and personal future? While public and professional discussion has not so far included anthropological knowledge within its consultative range, our commentary asks what contemporary social anthropology might add to these pressing debates. What might anthropological approaches have to offer?

The organisation and symbolism of predictive cultures are by no means novel subjects of ethnographic enquiry for social anthropologists. Ethnographic and historical analyses of divination and prophecy have recorded the special mediatory powers of medicine men, high priests, spiritualists, elders and others to interpret and avert both past and future misfortune.[7] Whether the scale of affliction is perceived as relatively circumscribed to a few persons' neglectful relations with ancestors, or manifest as a more extensive form of group-level suffering, divinatory processes all follow particular set routines by which otherwise inaccessible, or 'hidden', information is obtained by culturally accredited 'experts'. Because divination has been conceptualised as a mystical technique allied to magical [read 'primitive'] medicines, anthropologists of the structural-functionalist persuasion fell readily into slotting the concept of divination into the intellectualist perspective of the relative rationality of a given culture and its peoples.[8] However, drawing upon existing ethnographic data, there are a number of *limited* parallels one may ascertain between previous anthropological analysis of divination in non-Western cultures and the scientific cultures of prediction of early twenty-first century biotechnology.

Evans-Pritchard's (1937) seminal anthropological investigation of links between oracles, magic and manipulation among the Azande locates the power of revelatory effect at the corporeal level of the human body. In Zande divinatory practice, ordeals are likened to trials by divination whereby an accused person's *body* becomes the determinant of the unknown. In activating a form of socially innovative transformation, oracles require the performance of an experiment to determine the unknown (for instance the administration of *benge* substance to fowls).[9] The divination, then, is supposed to create a sense of certainty as to why things have happened; to reveal the truth as a kind of divinatory authority (Whyte 1991:165). Writing on forms of power and manipulation in Sierra Leone, especially the dynamics of Temne divinatory knowledge, anthropologist Rosalind Shaw suggests that the 'divisions of oracular labour' involve a truth-constructing process that leads to a *'public reclassification of people and events'* (Shaw 1991:140, emphasis added). Like the 'decoding' practices of genomics that attempt to map the human genome by sequencing the formerly obscure and unknown DNA code (see Chapter 2), the temporal logics of divination combine the *techne* of revelation and concealment with that of manipulation and transformation (i.e. of divining tools, identities and bodies).

Note however this is not to say that genetics and divination *are* isomorphic practices, only that both deploy a set of practices as certain kinds of skill or *techne*. I am of course turning the anthropological tables somewhat and stretching the traditional meaning of the diviner's role as cultural innovator, at least as exemplified by certain area-specific ethnography. Diviners of course are ritual specialists whose interventions are usually made manifest as specific effects by way of a special mediating or intermediary object. The *yiteendi* for instance is a coin or small piece of cloth in the diviner's possession which, as the Yaka people of Zaire insist, must have been in physical contact already with the aggrieved person who is making a claim against a past affliction (Devisch 1991). As I am intimating however, it is also possible to see in the person of the social anthropologist a mediating relation and intermediary object that moves between the domains of 'science' and 'ethics'. In the particular British context pursued here, describing and theorising the morality of divination turns specifically around the sociality of the pre-emptively 'pre-symptomatic' (or 'pre-dispositional') person. For our purposes the important point to stress is that a diverse panoply of ritual objects, omens, acts, expert cosmological or religious knowledge may be brought skilfully into conjunction, or deployed on its own, as *mediumistic guides for future action*. Oracles, in this sense, constitute a kind of experimental (material) technology of manipulation, not altogether unlike certain Western discourses or instruments that are said to characterise the innovations of modern 'science in action' (e.g. Galison and Stump 1996).

In her analysis of the genetic reading of breast screening 'omens', medical anthropologist Margaret Lock (1998) discusses the relationship between oracles and manipulation not simply in terms of concrete laboratory techniques and other material practices, but according to how scientists elide the discourse of risk with the abstraction of probability. Lock argues first that the new technology of genetic testing is an example of a divination practice that links the individual to the past, namely one's genetic inheritance, and reinforces interest in the interpretation of future 'omens' in the context of soliciting the likelihood of becoming ill in the future.[10] She quotes Evans-Pritchard's remark that '... when the oracles announce that a man will fall sick ... his "condition" is therefore already bad, *his future is already part of him*' (Lock 1998:7, emphasis added). The second part of Lock's argument, derived from Hacking's (1990) thesis on constructs of chance, concerns the taming of probability through the creation of a new category of risk. Lock here highlights how it is not just bodies that are (genetically) manipulated, but chance itself.[11] She rightly points to discrepancies between official science statistics (for instance penetrance rates and abstract, reified 'at risk' beliefs) and the actual experience of particular cases of any given individual.[12] In particular, Lock carefully unravels some of the consequences of failing to pay attention to epidemiological inconstants that are based on the 'premature transformation of "possible" probabilities ... into "certain" probabilities' (Lock 1998: 13).

> Diviners are usually careful not to make extravagant claims about the management of omens ... Today, however, certain interested parties forge ahead under the twin banners of probability theory and molecular genetics, offering certainty and control through the manipulation of genes *(ibid)*.

Now, instead of basing these cross-cultural divination and revelation comparisons around a discursive interlacing of magic, science and practical activity[13] it would seem more fruitful to assert a shift from questions of rationality altogether, to ones that critique concepts of morality through the semantic register of divination. So far as the Western context goes, I suggest this to be a matter of charting an analytical shift from the conventional primacy of the informational idiom (and associated forms of biological reductionism) to the morality of divination as *ethno-ethical* knowledge (see section below). The comments of anthropologist Philip Peek (1991) are particularly helpful here. Peek remarks that the study of divination needs to be explored in the larger context of decision-making in everyday life and not simply in terms of religious phenomena (Peek 1991:13). Seen as an anthropological tool for establishing comparative epistemology, this broadened ideational remit values the concept of divination as a source of knowledge-in-action; as a dynamic system upon which the ordering of social action is based as a creative means of decision-making.

Ethno-ethics and the encounter with biology

I begin by way of a provocation. This is simply to make the observation that social and medical anthropologists generally have not taken the disciplinary lead in initiating a conceptual and methodological agenda to which bioethicists might be roused to respond. Nonetheless there are compelling reasons why contemporary anthropology might be more proactive in seeking to devise such a programme at just this point in time. Aside from the specifics of predictive genetics, debates about 'health ethics imperialism' involving clinical research between 'sponsor' and 'host' countries as well as other developments in global health and human rights more generally (see e.g. Benatar 1998) invite critical reconstruction of the field of 'bio-ethics' as a *cultural* phenomenon in its own right.

Richard Lieban's (1990) proposal to develop an 'ethno-ethics' to explore cross-cultural variation in international health seems particularly suggestive. Lieban suggests that the study of comparative medical moralities need not be limited to a reckoning of differences between ostensibly separate cultures, but that the value of ethno-ethical information lies partly in terms of the analyst's ability to establish points of contact as cross-cultural ethical similarities. An ethnoethics agenda 'should contribute to the discourse on medical ethics not only by illuminating culturally distinctive moral views and problems, but also by helping to provide *a more realistic and knowledgeable basis for the exploration of cross-cultural ethical similarities*' (Lieban 1990:223, emphasis added). This can be taken as an invitation to explore ethics as yet another 'belief' system in need of critical anthropological analysis. Anthropologists might wish to experiment to see how a comparative 'ethno-ethics' can be turned back upon the West so as to reconsider the value of a bioethics framework in terms of its own originating context. Insofar as the discursive production of *genethics* is very obviously an artefact of Western moral sensibility, it too lends itself to critical scrutiny according to this ethno-ethical imperative (see Chapter 2). Part of the aim of this book is to see how the solicitous deployment of comparative materials sets up the possibility to pursue a number of conceptual cross-linkages between diverse cultural experiences without violating the specifics of a given case. Ethno-ethics for our purposes is a linked analytic endeavour dependent on the application of theory (Singer 1992) as a 'narrative ethics'. One of the strengths and still relatively unexplored dimensions of narrative analysis is the potential to locate theories *in* the narration of practices rather than as abstract values necessarily underlying them. Witness the way that recent work in medical anthropology, for instance, documents stories of sickness by examining moral dilemmas within a biographical framework (Frank 2000; Mattingly 1998; Skultans 2000; Ingstad and Whyte 1995). The narratives pertaining to 'genome stories' are more complicated methodological agendas because 'persons' may take beguiling forms in which they are not always self-evident as conscious or intentional moral agents. Specifically there are the ambiguous social entities of the embryo and pre-embryo. Now whether one is exploring the cultural selection processes of pre-conceptive technologies, or whether value is negotiated in terms of the 'pre-symptomatic' person's status as new classificatory knowledge, attending to processes of reasoning may mean deflecting one's gaze away from an exclusive focus on abstracted ideals. As medical anthropologist Arthur Kleinman (1995:67) explains:

> The cardinal contribution of the anthropologist of medicine to bioethics . . . is to deeply humanize *the process of formulating an ethical problem* by allowing variation and pluralism and the constraints of social positions to emerge and receive their due, so that ethical standards are not imposed in an alien and authoritarian way but, rather, are actualised as the outcome of reciprocal participatory engagement across different worlds of experience (emphasis added).

This appeal to participatory engagement across different worlds of experience invites a broad and rich conceptualisation of 'bioethics' that is not only sensitive to the lived experience of families – the ordinary man or woman – but explicitly interdisciplinary or integrative in its aims (see Chapter 2). If narrating the lived experience of families can contribute to a rewriting of the grounds of medical authority and 'expertise', then so-called 'narrative ethics' is also about the many difficult and uncertain moments the ethnographer undergoes in the processes of story telling itself.[14] It is about the moral reasoning by which the story teller is able to make the narrative at all possible or plausible as an account in its own right.

Narrating Huntington's Disease families

Huntington's Disease (HD) was the first neuro-degenerative condition for which predictive genetic tests became available in the late 1980s. It is a rare monogenic (single-gene) disorder of the central nervous system characterised by involuntary movements and progressive dementia, for which, at present, there is no known available cure. Though worldwide figures have been hard to compile, it is estimated that about one person in every 10,000 is affected in the UK (see Harper 1996). The condition usually affects adults in mid-life, though sometimes manifests in childhood, and for this reason is loosely referred to as a 'late-onset' illness. A progressive disease lasting anything from ten to twenty years or longer, affected persons may experience a range of ongoing personality changes such as impulsive, forgetful, depressive or violent behaviour. In physical terms one suffers from gradual loss of speech and general deterioration of reflexes to the point where swallowing becomes so difficult that choking is a frequent cause of death. Although symptoms of the illness are not evident at birth, it is a condition that is genetically transmitted from parent to child in a pattern known as 'autosomal dominant' inheritance, meaning that only one parent of either sex need have the disorder to pass it on to genetically related offspring. Clinicians routinely refer to this in terms of the probability of offspring of an affected individual having a 50 per cent chance of inheriting the disease (see Cox and McKellin 1999), a way of thinking – as we will see – that is quite different to subjects' own pre-symptomatic illness narratives.

Pre-symptomatic testing for HD has been available to families from 1986, at first using linkage analysis based on the genetic comparison of blood samples taken from the various family members of a genetic test candidate or 'proband', based upon the analysis of medical pedigrees.[15] Following the successful identification in 1993 of the gene mutation associated with HD (see Huntington's Disease Collaborative Research Group 1993) a definitive or 'direct' predictive test has been possible for self-selecting individuals.[16] In contrast with linkage testing, the direct test is based upon analysis of the region of DNA implicated in the activation of the disease. This region, located on the short arm of chromosome 4, is characterised by the long stretch of polyglutamine present in HD protein, and is referred to in clinical terms as the expansion of the trinucleotide sequence of CAG bases (see Harper 1996).[17]

Fortunately not everyone who goes for genetic testing will face such a bleak prognosis as members of the HD population. Yet in a world in which growing numbers of disorders may be diagnosed before symptoms appear, even though there may be no effective therapy for them, the response of the HD community, though not necessarily paradigmatic, certainly holds out strong interest. In the early spring of 1998 I started to meet with members and activists from the HD community, many of whom were affiliated to several of the regional branches of the UK national support organisation, the Huntington's Disease Association (HDA), or had previously attended the Association's Annual Conference event. Upon first meeting HD-affected families I was intrigued by the way people would describe their lives as living pre-symptomatic time and what this meant for carriers with positive test results and their relations with untested kin. It had struck me already, well before I commenced by own field research, that the genetic knowledge acquired in these situations was 'information' of a very specific kind. Those who took the test clearly received no accurate prognosis as to when exactly they would start to become ill. And so it was largely from the vagueness of this observation that I set out to study how genomic science enjoins a new ethics of classificatory knowledge relating to the moral sensibilities and categorisation of persons who have been identified as 'pre-ill' before they are 'ill'. In terms of staging an ethnographic encounter, I became immersed in practices relating to the emergence of 'at risk' populations, noting how a new class of 'pre-symptomatic' persons, based around the consciousness of a pre-emptive diagnostic rationality, changed people's everyday lives and social relations. After presenting the aims of my study to regular members of HD support groups, this period of fieldwork relied upon intensive repeat home interviews. I got to know particular families well by joining in certain of their HD fundraising activities such as sponsored walks, and was fortunate to be invited to attend other HD-organised social events such as home barbecues and birthday parties. Spending time at patient support groups, user forums and meetings, participating in local branch meetings and holding numerous conversations with regional care advisers, I was able to build up close familiarity with forty-six individuals from twenty-two separate households all of whom took part as voluntary 'interlocutors' in intensive semi-structured and unstructured interviews. Interviewees contributing to this research study may be further sub-divided in terms of:

(1) Those confirmed as 'at risk' after receipt of a positive predictive test result.
(2) Those who were potentially pre-symptomatic (with knowledge of a familial hereditary transmission) and whose risk had been removed through a negative test result.
(3) Those married to persons known to be at risk or confirmed pre-symptomatic (abbreviated as HD in-marrying partners).
(4) In-marrying partners who have knowledge of the familial illness prior to conjugal relations (a sub-group of particular interest from the point of view of family planning and pre-implantation genetic diagnosis exclusion techniques).

(5) In-marrying partners who unexpectedly learn 'out of the blue' about a family in-law's/spouses's HD predicament.
(6) Offspring as descendants of the affected.
(7) Other first-degree relatives of the affected, including siblings, cousins, uncles, aunts, parents, grandparents.[18]

At the outset of my fieldwork I had also just read *Mapping Fate*, Alice Wexler's (1996) detailed and intimate personal memoir of her own family's HD geneal-ogy in which the author retraces her mother's slow deterioration and eventual death against the wider research backdrop of international science collabo-rations. Wexler chronicles how the clinical dream of developing a predictive genetic test, long cherished by geneticists and counsellors, as well as by many affected families, eventually became a reality thanks in no small part to the tireless campaigning efforts of her sister and father, Nancy and Milton Wexler. Since the late 1960s, the Wexler family had played a pivotal role in the organ-isation and sponsorship of genetic research in the United States through the Heredity Disease Foundation, the organisation the family had established and to which they had dedicated most of their professional lives (see Wexler 1979, 1992). Wexler's account struck me for its honesty, both in charting the Wexler sisters' own relation to living with an 'at risk' identity, and for the author's open ambivalence about how to write a critical account of these past scientific developments without jeopardising the future of genetic research in this area. As Wexler's authorial voice assumed critical resonance and distanced itself from members of her birth family, and indeed the wider science community, Wexler concerned herself with all the usual sorts of self-presentation problems that consume much ethnographic research practice as well as the reflexive pro-cesses of writing. Whose voice may be heard? Whose speech is legitimate? Who can tell their own story when it also involves the stories of others? For whom and to what ends is new knowledge being written? What ought not to get written? Since *Mapping Fate* unfolds as a narrative journey that explores both sisters' increasing ambivalence towards the revelations of genetic prophecy, it is also a story about finding a position from which to articulate the meaning and value of non-knowledge. Alice and Nancy's decisions not to take the predictive test transformed Wexler's story into an autobiography that is 'less about an ill-ness than about *the possibility* of an illness, less about the medical dilemma of living with disease than about the existential dilemma of living at risk' (Wexler 1996:xxii, emphasis added).[19]

Already from these initial observations it seemed to me that the distance between the power of scientists to predict diseases and their limited ability to cure or treat them called for much closer ethnographic scrutiny. Similarly one could hardly dismiss the fact that across Western Europe clinicians themselves were also starting to report evidence of a much lower uptake of pre-symptomatic tests for HD than had been expected prior to the development of the predictive test. In the absence of effective therapy, statistics from several studies revealed that far fewer people were opting to take the test (see Meissen and Berchek 1987; Craufurd *et al.* 1989; Tibbens *et al.* 1992). Turning to Wexler's 'confessions', these seemed to me to look more like a grass-roots account of the uncertain deliberations of how best to deal with genetic foreknowledge as a form of prognostic morality (see Chapter 3). From this perspective, it is important to explore not just why people might be refusing to come forward and take the test, but how those who did decide to do so subsequently went on to define themselves as 'pre-symptomatic'. Since so little is known in general about how kin make moral decisions about health outside the confines of the clinical setting, it is important to chart how the acquisition of new genetic knowledge through such 'revelatory' predictions may change one's sense of self and associated notions of well being. What, in other words, does it really mean to be 'pre-symptomatic'?

Whilst much academic literature on the ethics of genetic testing acknowledges that the decision whether or not to be tested for 'late-onset' illness poses major life dilemmas for pre-symptomatic individuals,[20] only a handful of studies in the social sciences consider the impacts of predictive genetic testing on changing conceptions of the family and ideas about human relatedness more generally.[21] The particular aim of this book is to explore how affected and non-affected kin, as divergent moral agents, encounter and negotiate their status as 'pre-symptomatic' persons and as inter-generational relations. In other words, it is the specific choices that people make that are explored here: the cultural imaginary supporting the worlds of the 'pre-symptomatic'. Let me clarify what is meant here by the term 'cultural imaginary'. The term 'culture' is not deployed in this book as a referent simply collapsible with ethnic or cultural difference, as medical categorisation and rationale so commonly assume. What the anthropologist as diviner is likely to be particularly interested in is the link 'culture' allows to be made between that which is non-visible and that which is recognised as 'a-symptomatic' or 'pre-symptomatic'. Some of the questions and issues stemming from this interest bear upon the following dilemmas: what does it mean to have the knowledge that one's body harbours the deferred and not yet visible symptoms of a 'late-onset' illness? What does it mean to have this susceptibility made explicit? In these contexts, I would suggest that 'culture' refers to the analytic work that bridges a link between the categories of 'disease' and 'person' where both seem to be connected by the paradox *neither* may be defined in terms of manifest illness, nor for that matter, available remedy.

'Culture' is put to work, then, in terms of the apparent rationalisation that whilst the testing of genes provides a prognosis, it fails resolutely – at least for the present – to provide a cure. How people live this paradox, strive to derive meaning and create sense from, as well as evade the effects of the new life technologies, are all vital questions for ethnographic study given the prospect of a future era of genetic governmentality. For anthropology, not only relaying these findings to a non-anthropological audience but also seeking actively to create sites of potential collaboration with clinical geneticists, health professionals, bioethicists and others, is all part of the ongoing task of 'translocating' culture.

Organisation of the book

Although the chapters each look at different aspects of the status of genetic information and the cultural implications of creating new kinds of genetic knowledge, each may be read as interlinked sites that explore the relationship between genetic testing technologies and the making of the pre-symptomatic person. Unravelling the contours of a critical ethnography, our focus will be guided conceptually by a series of 'translocations'. These translocations trace opportunities for the creative mixing of particular thought styles informing certain conventions within the natural and social sciences. Chapter 2, 'Approaching translocations', is an extended conceptual analysis of the interdisciplinary relations between ethics, ethnography and the science of genetics. In classical Mendelian genetics, 'translocation' describes what happens when a fragment of one chromosome sporadically and accidentally breaks off and becomes attached to a different chromosome, either in a somatic cell or while a gamete is being made during fertilisation. In other words, translocation refers to what can go wrong and defy 'nature' during the process of crossing over between different parental sets of chromosomes at meiosis. Insisting on the mutual processes of creativity that can come from juxtaposing different, and usually separated, orders of knowledge, here the practice of ethnography is shown to borrow, and again to modify the concept of 'linkage map', a term traditionally associated with the natural process of DNA 'recombination'.

Such discursive exchange between the disciplines seeks to redesign the landscape of human biology outside of the long-standing Westernised dichotomies of nature-culture. The guiding theme of translocations, as an analytical framework for the subsequent chapters, probes the possibility of simultaneously crossing continents and crossing chromosomes as critical integrative exploration – it is a local instantiation of 'ethno-ethics'. From this the relationship between genes, human embodiment and moral knowledge may be charted as kinds of holistic 'lifelines' (cf. Rose 1997).

In Part II we shift to the intimate specifics of family life. Chapters 3–6, based on fieldwork and in-depth case studies of some six families affected by Huntington's Disease, comprise the heart of the ethnographic enterprise. Here we are concerned with the generation and narration of particular 'home truths'. We consider how these truths are elicited as processes of value construction within local moral worlds of genetic prognostication. Where newly acquired knowledge of a late-onset genetically inherited illness becomes a part of every-day reality for a given family, cross-generational and inter-generational relations between kin are seen to be affected in a number of ways. The test result, and the 'revelation' it brings for people, is seen to be a life-transforming event, but it is one that cannot simply be localised to the space of the clinic, nor confined to the time of the present. Once a predictive test result has been delivered as a new predispositional 'truth', and once the clinician and the testee go their separate ways, how does such genetic knowledge transform persons as the substance of ethical relations? Chapter 3, 'Foretelling foreknowledge', examines in depth how people describe their experiences of anticipating future illness, both before and after the oracular 'revelations' of genetic testing. It shows how the eval-uative criteria, the 'diagnostic' and 'predictive' tools through which medical science attempts to classify people, are at odds with the way individuals and families over time provisionally 'test out', and painfully make sense of, their own uncertain worlds of prophetic genetics.

Chapter 4, 'Tracing genealogies of non-disclosure', juxtaposes the dilemmas of truth telling informing conventional bioethics on the one hand, with infor-mants' own views of the liabilities of veracity on the other. We look at how issues of concealment and non-knowledge frame many of these pre-symptomatic ill-ness narratives, and situate the discussion in the wider context of certain contem-porary policy debates. Particular attention is paid to the bioethical principle of 'unsolicited disclosure' and the emotionality relating to breaches of disclosure. Does a person violate a kin's assumed right not to know genetic information by disclosing certain knowledge? Does a person violate a relative's assumed right to information about their health by not saying anything? How are children included in decisions about genetic testing? How are these dilemmas changing concepts of relatedness?

The inter-generational transmission of genetic (non) knowledge, especially the parental dilemmas of 'telling' children they may be 'at risk', as well as the upwards flows of knowledge whereby positively tested children necessarily implicate their (untested) parents, raise important cultural questions about the meaning of individual claims to privacy and confidentiality. By drawing out the ethico-temporal aspects of new genealogical knowledge, the chapter builds up a base from which it is possible to discuss a relational model of ethical

reflexivity that challenges certain assumptions of mainstream bioethics. It also
introduces a range of comparative materials from the medical anthropological literature. By drawing selectively upon certain ethnographic materials such
as Murray Last's work on Hausa medical culture, Cecilia McCallum's analysis of the links between health and embodied agency among the Amazonian
Cashinahua and Gilbert Lewis's work on illness revelation among the Gnau
people of West Sepik province, Papua New Guinea, this comparative focus
serves as critical relief for the 'right to know' debates of Western bioethical
discourse (e.g., Chadwick *et al.* 1997). These ethnographic materials illustrate
how constructs of personhood may be conceived as the negotiated embodiment
of moral knowledge in situations of illness and health adversity.

Chapters 5 and 6 go on to explore changing perceptions and idioms of
heredity. In Chapter 5 'Reproducing exclusion', we look more closely at same
generational relations to show how conflicts of interest over claims to genetic
knowledge between family members do not always divide simply along exclusively genetic lines. The theme of exclusion is carried forward once more in
Chapter 6 in order to explore the ethical dilemmas and decision-making processes relating to developments in pre-conceptive 'reprogenetic' technologies.
'Relinquishing exclusion' considers the technique of pre-implantation genetic
diagnosis (PGD) and the temporal dynamics that shape genetic knowledge in
these procreative contexts of foreknowledge. By making it possible for prospective parents with a known hereditary disorder such as HD to decide which of
their in-vitro fertilised embryo(s) they wish to have implanted, such embryos,
as potential forms of life, become 'pre-symptomatic' entities before they are
even born. We see on the one hand that Darwinian and sociobiological notions
of 'natural selection' and 'kin selection' are rendered anachronistic conceptions given the newly extended repertoire of technological choice. On the other,
prospective parents' decisions to withhold kinship exclusion through the *non-
termination* of a pregnancy comprise instances of 'cultural selectionism'. This
chapter offers, then, an early indicative picture of some ways that mothers and
fathers are refusing on certain occasions the values of an incipient 'new eugenicist' agenda. As a concluding statement, the final chapter brings together the
main themes of the book and places many of the case studies and theoretical
discussion within the wider context of debates about predictive biofutures and
the biopolitics of cure. By taking apart the different meanings, inflections and
embodied experiences of living 'pre-symptomatically' and by situating these
examples within specified contexts, I argue that the term is likely to remain
powerfully ambiguous for both social practice and critical analysis.

2

Approaching translocations

Cross-talking value

In a large conference hall in the district of Fontenoy, Paris, representatives from eighty-one nation states from all corners of the world were busy deliberating official reports concerning you, me and the futures of countless other human beings. It was the last week in July 1997 and a Committee of Governmental Experts convened by UNESCO and supported by members of its International Bioethics Committee (IBC), was in the process of adopting the ninth and final draft of the Universal Declaration on the Human Genome and Human Rights.[1]

In the opening and closing addresses to the meeting, Federico Mayer, the then Director-General and his colleague Héctor Gros Espiell, sought to clarify the instrumental status of the Declaration. Though its contents could effect no legal binding force, both speakers reminded committee participants of the need to reach an ethical framework for human genome practice that would concur with 'principles of a durable nature'.[2] Taken in its entirety the Declaration may indeed be read as the formal 'story' of how science and ethics have met directly through the universal kinship figure of the human genome. The opening article states that the human genome is the symbolic 'heritage of humanity' and encompasses 'the fundamental unity of all members of the human family, as well as the recognition of their inherent dignity and diversity'. A couple of paragraphs later in a section devoted to the prescriptive checks and balance of scientific progress, we learn that no research or technological applications concerning the genome should prevail over respect for human rights, fundamental freedoms and the dignity of persons.

What, one might ask, do such high-minded statements (coming from such a source) reveal about political process and the negotiation of value differences relevant to science and health in a multicultural world? Aware of the far-ranging implications of developments in the life and health sciences, in

particular genetics and molecular biology, UNESCO had formally endorsed
the currency of 'bioethics' as the conceptual basis of a legitimate transcultural
debate. It was the framework of a shared bioethics agenda that was seen as
capable of governing and transcending the divisions of spatial borders and cultural difference. The international community, it was felt, could be enlisted not
simply as an abstract ideal but in actual practice through the consensual activity
of committee experts doing the business of ethico-political codification.[3]

Now while signatories to the Declaration appeared to agree to many concepts and principles, for onlookers it seems both hopeful and surprising that
heads of state and their representatives should have converged so seamlessly
across the extensive fields of biology, genetics and medicine.[4] Sceptics of a
genuine cross-cultural consensus might point out certain limiting constraints,
and cultural anthropologists interested in the practical and theoretical possibilities for a modelling of trans-cultural ethics would be naturally attentive to these
developments. For one thing, the human genome itself and the very epistemic
practice of molecular biology it emanates, happens to be a specific historical
product of Western scientific invention, funding and institutional collaboration. The cultural imaginary of progress that genome research both signifies
and supports is at odds with many non-Western conceptions of human origins,
human and non-human interdependencies, notions of well being and diverse
cross-cultural beliefs about the efficacy of indigenous forms of healing. Since
the Drafting Committee condensed the report of its mediatory work into just
two and a half pages, it is difficult to convey how and indeed the extent to
which cross-regional differences were deliberated, nor how these differences
were tentatively resolved during the deliberation process, let alone linguistically
translated.[5] What we can surmise from a reading of the relevant sections of the
Final Report is evidence of internal disagreement relating to the concept of 'the
human genome as the common heritage of humanity'. This wording was finally
amended to 'the heritage of humanity', and in stressing the symbolic value of
the heritage notion as distinct from an exclusively materialist legacy, members
hoped to preclude potential abuse of the genome through collective forms of
appropriation (UNESCO 1997a:9). Less clear though were the kinds of belief
and values that led representatives overwhelmingly to reject the attribution of
'common' as a descriptive referent for the (universal) human genome. What was
the Drafting Committee excluding in its version of these ostensibly historical
events in genome ethics?

Since I open with an example from the United Nations, I should stress that
this book is not about the international politics of postgenomic science. Nor is
it an apology or critique of the 'epistemic charity' of Western science, a theme
pursued by such science and culture theorists as Meera Nanda, Ziauddin Sardar

and Susantha Goonatilake, for example. It is, however, an exercise in integrative biology that endeavours to ask how a comparative anthropology can begin to conceptualise an ethno-ethical framework of potential relevance to certain aspects of contemporary genomics (see Chapter 1). As such it represents a *parallel* but separate venture to global bioethics initiatives such as the current WHO Human Genetics Programme and its particular rationales informing local 'ethical' involvement in various parts of the developing world (WHO 2002). As a happily vexed 'halfie' anthropologist witnessing indigenous developments in genetic science from the perspective of contemporary biomedical Britain, this particular exercise in 'home-work' entails ongoing instruction in certain processes of unlearning and deep ambivalence. Favourite lessons are not only those that disrupt home/exoticist distributions of knowledge but ones that reorient at the same time the spatial organisation of the observing fieldworker as primary witness to new temporal sensibilities.[6]

Well, taking the liberty to conjecture . . . What the various signatories may have imagined they shared was less a belief about the cultural value of the entity of the human genome *per se* than a common sense that old dichotomies between notions of 'traditional' and 'modern' were slipping away for everyone alike. More precisely, previous distinctions between so-called 'small-scale' and industrialised 'complex' societies seen as the difference between orientations towards cyclical and linear time – at least so far as an earlier anthropological imagination is concerned – dissolved into the awareness of an interconnected community getting 'locked into' new futures. I don't mean to sound deterministic here, only to signal a rupture in distinctions between reversible and irreversible valuations of time and what an anthropological eye might previously have imagined as the structural taxonomy of 'hot' and 'cold' societies. The metaphors hold good even today though appear to come attached with a different set of symbolic referents.

'Hot' science, 'cold' ethics?

Ever since the early modern period and the European Enlightenment of the late seventeenth century, the relationship between scientific facts and social values has been an uneasy one. As most schoolchildren introduced to the history of Western science will learn, Galileo Galilei came to blows with his Jesuit inquisitors because he refused to accept the compatibility of Copernicus's sun-centred universe and the Bible. While today's secular science imputes value to domains other than religion, many Western scientists and ethicists continue to defend their respective fields of knowledge as though they denote mutually exclusive spheres of practice and belief. The conventional view holds that Western science extols itself as the domain of objective 'fact' with direct access to an external order and context-independent truth; ethics meanwhile concerns the faculty of moral judgement predicated upon notions of human 'value'. Facts may be gleaned by carefully controlled observation capable of precise quantification and unambiguous expression. Value categories on the other hand do not form any one-to-one correspondence with 'natural' categories, and, unlike the organised pursuit of scientific knowledge, cannot be analysed independently of other social practice.

This scientistic gloss on the fact-value distinction perpetuates yet another self-serving ideological 'truth': the view that the 'cold' study of ethics lags behind the 'hot' advances of science. Ethical policy and theory, as a form of reasoning about scientific progress has evolved out of concerns over the 'right' and 'wrong' way to apply new knowledge; it is not fundamentally an inventive force in its own right but simply responsive to past scientific inventions, developments or imminent 'breakthroughs'. This particular belief, extensively promoted by scientists, is intimately bound up with certain conceptions about what distinguishes 'good' science from 'bad' science. The 'truth squads' that inflamed the Anglophone 'science wars' in the 1990s amidst Alan Sokal's famous hoax and attack upon what he and other scientists saw as the 'glib relativism' of much cultural studies of science, was not just a conflict *between* academic cultures.[7] It was also the continuation of a running commentary on the embeddedness of science in society that stoked pre-existing internal science disputes about the morality of science, especially its relation to concepts of 'value'. At stake has been the political question of different kinds of scientific accountability. So-called 'objectivist' scientists continue to promote a view of 'good' science by arguing that the validity of moral principles cannot be inferred from the factual discoveries of science (the view that an 'ought' cannot be derived from an 'is'). They are countered by 'normative' scientists, the more vocal of whom may suggest that a scientist's 'true' scientific belief coincides with ethically acceptable social effects.[8]

In one of his last works, the palaeontologist and popular science writer Stephen Jay Gould attempted to level out these science and anti-science binarisms with his exegesis of the two metaphorical 'rocks of ages': 'to cite the old clichés' Gould remarks, 'science gets the age of rocks, and religion the rock of ages' (Gould 2001:6). These equivalences aside, this imagery of permanence configures also some intriguing conceptual work. The 'rocks of ages' serve further as a rhetorical device for Gould's thesis of 'non-overlapping magisteria', the principle of NOMA. A magisterium, he observes, is 'a domain where one form of teaching holds the appropriate tools for meaningful discourse and resolution' (*ibid*, 5), and though there are many such domains, two principal exemplars are the magisterium of scientific inquiry and the magisterium of ethics and values.

If we look further into the NOMA concept, we see that it works strategically as a way of bringing together two usually discrete premises in mainstream Western science talk. Gould is insisting that science and ethics comprise two 'different but equally vital' endeavours (*ibid*, 53). The political point expressed here is that the binarisms between science and non-science represent false conflicts of war, and that NOMA is a tactic for 'respectful non-interference' that encourages 'supportive dialogue' between the magisteria. Thus, Gould observes that:

> Science and religion do not glower at each other from separate frames on opposite walls of the Museum of Mental Arts. Science and religion interdigitate in patterns of complex fingering, and at every fractal scale of self-similarity (65).

Energised by NOMA's potential capacities for 'resolution' this is Gould's conciliatory, and for some, plainly idealistic vision. However, as Gould himself admits in the book's opening sentence, the NOMA concept is in fact 'blessedly simple and *entirely conventional*' (Gould 2001: 3, emphasis added). In insisting that these magisteria comprise specifically 'non-overlapping' domains, Gould retreats to a stance that relocates the power of science in terms of its conventional epistemological autonomy (as summed up in the designation of Mode I Science in Nowotny *et al.* [2002]). Immediately after the appeal to 'interdigitated' form, there is retraction in the very next sentence with its admission magisteria do not overlap. Gould may well have creditable intentions in impressing that different disciplinary knowledge cannot be joined together in any kind of grand intellectual synthesis. However, the interplay between interdigitation and the view that boundaries between fields of knowledge can be separated neatly so as to leave only discrete auto-referential systems reinstates the beliefs of the objectivists mentioned above. Ultimately Gould here is saying nothing new: indeed throughout his tract we hear the familiar refrain that science is to be left 'entirely free in its own proper magisterium' and 'science rules the magisterium of factual truth about nature' (22).

Do we really have to go on with these 'warfare' models of knowledge and knowledge production? Are we still at the start of the new millennium, so fixed in a dichotomous 'two cultures' mindset that we cannot think ourselves out of C. P. Snow's famous formulation? Are non-overlapping magisteria as good as it gets, and is ethics in Western cultures always simply reducible to the norms of good and bad – and the related hot and cold polarities of relative progress? It is beyond the scope of the present book to answer all these questions in any satisfactory depth. But by exploring how ethnography can traverse ethics and science as a relation of mediation and critical practice of translation, the relevance of cross-talking value may be seen to be stirring as an alternative conceptual direction.

Yet Gould is more interesting than my commentary would suggest. Although he gives a wide berth to the content of the 'turf' disputes that characterised the 'science wars' – mainly on the grounds that these are, as he claims, fictional factions – he does actually want to say something engaging about culture. 'The magisterium of science', he notes, '*cannot proceed beyond the anthropology of morals*' (Gould 2001:65, emphasis added). There are at least two ways of reading this. As a statement of limits, the claim serves to draw certain boundaries between fact and speculation, between a factual 'is' and an ethical 'ought'. The magisterium of science, the statement suggests, cannot base itself on the comparative study of morals. We may be able to prove that most Euro-Americans believe that eating people is wrong but that does not mean we can prove that eating people *is* wrong. In other words, it is not possible to derive an 'ought' from the reckoning of what 'is'. Relativist and pluralist positions in social anthropology would happily go along with this, but Gould writing from the perspective of the evolutionary biologist happens to have a rather specific view of what he thinks constitutes an anthropology of morals as a viable field of cultural study. The full length of Gould's sentence reads as follows:

> The magisterium of science cannot proceed beyond the anthropology of morals – the documentation of what people believe, including such important information as the relative frequency of particular moral values among distinct cultures, the correlation of those values with ecological and economic conditions, and even (potentially) the adaptive value of certain beliefs in specified Darwinian situations (*ibid*).

Gould is repeating the once classic anthropological quest for pure tradition and discrete cultural difference, and mixing into this anachronistic ideal the ethnocentric speculations of a Darwinian biology. Implicitly, the magisterium of science cannot proceed beyond an anthropology of morals because moral accountability cannot drive a theory of ethics over and beyond the remit of positivist fact. In other words, Gould's innocent looking one-liner condenses a view of ethics as flaccid and 'cold'. The other more charitable way of reading the statement is to see an anthropology of morality as the epistemological mover arbitrating the meaning of value itself. In which case, science cannot proceed beyond the cross-cultural study of morality because anthropology has something interesting to say *to* science and science should take note! In either case, just look how easy it is for the scientist to cross into anthropology and appear to make authoritative judgements about the status of moral ethnography! But let's assume Gould is waving a welcoming signal to fellow humanities. How then does socio-cultural anthropology respond?

Anthropology, ethics and bioethics

It was Raymond Firth who first pointed out in his Marett Lecture in 1953 that comparative analysis of the cultural parameters of 'value' as a key conceptual referent of anthropological analysis has been uneven, unsystematic and mainly descriptive. Though much early social anthropology did investigate the normative behaviour and moral codes of different cultures, it is only relatively recently that the comparative study of culture as moral action has roused renewed theoretical interest in the subject of indigenous *moralities* (e.g. Fluehr-Lobban 2003; Caplan 2003; Laidlaw 2002; Faubion 2002; Strathern 2000). As Howell (1997:5) observes, it would be helpful to 'identify as many arenas as possible which may serve as 'pegs' for analysis for future anthropological studies of moralities'. In the light of this renewed focus, the mid-century empirical interest in the anthropological study of 'values' (witness, *inter alia*, Read 1955; Edel and Edel 1959; Kluckhohn and Strodtbeck 1961) is often forgotten. In part this is attributable to the fact that no separate domain came to be carved out as a relevant disciplinary sub-division for the systematic study of 'ethics'. It is also because 'the locus of the 'moral', when it has been identified in anthropological writing, has too often been the morphology of convention itself, inevitably congruent with the forms of explicitly encoded religion, law, kinship, or whatever' (James 1988:144). So, despite the post-modernist turn away from normative social structure, little anthropological theory on the subject of morality had emerged in the 1980s – though not for want of critical articulation by a few defining voices. David Parkin's (1985) cross-cultural volume on evil identified not only the creativity of morality for social relations, but also the tendency of much anthropological analysis to avoid turning the fruits of its descriptive ethnographic endeavours into a critical conceptual arena for further theoretical examination of morality. Similarly, David Pocock (1986:7) was to note that the general neglect of ethics by anthropologists ought to make the discipline's academic practitioners 'downright embarrassed'.

But one early stab at theoretical exploration, following shortly on the heels of Kenneth Read's seminal paper on indigenous ethics amongst the Gahuku-Gama of the Eastern Highlands in Papua New Guinea, did represent a small test case in interdisciplinary collaborative venture. Though in many ways conceptually outmoded from today's vantage, May and Abraham Edel's (1968) *Anthropology and Ethics* remains something of a landmark in its attempt to bring together the respective insights of a social anthropologist and moral philosopher. Behind the united proposal to develop 'an anthropological transcription of ethical theory (1968:264), the analysis revealed some of the epistemic tensions between ethicists and anthropologists. Different disciplinary training, background and interests all played their part and could not be easily erased. In fairly general terms, moral philosophy deals with rule-based universal ethical propositions whose value inheres in the centrality of justification. The justification of moral judgements proceeds by subsuming facts under principles and rules, but as philosopher Barry Hoffmaster (1990:257) notes, 'principlism' is stymied in its own auto-referential trap: 'positivist morality so subordinates the descriptive that its 'justification' becomes justification in the abstract, which ultimately is no justification at all'. By abstracting cultural contexts and neglecting concrete experiential evidence, the concept of 'culture' in such analyses is either crudely caricatured for the extreme fracturing effects of cultural relativism, glossed as shared beliefs – usually synonymous with collective values – or else simply dispensed with altogether.[9] Where philosophy fails to recognise that the process of ethical deliberation is itself contextual and emergent, anthropology *may* tend towards excessive descriptive and contextual detail. In the past, this has led to an under-privileging of the development of theoretical critique during the analytical process of ethnographic research and exegesis. The production of ethnography has not been deployed *primarily* as theoretical exemplar, precedent or preferred conceptual tool, and so far as moral conceptual analysis goes, the primacy of rich description in anthropology has downplayed philosophical rumination as a mode of analytical reflection (see again Parkin 1985; also Pocock 1986).[10] There are of course exceptions. Caroline Humphrey's (1997) account of 'exemplary morality' finds sufficient descriptive and theoretical reason in the Mongolian cultivation of the self to question the European ethical ideal of harmonious resolution as part of a wider anthropological critique.

When one turns to recent debates about the under-development of theory in medical anthropology, it is the 'rules of engagement' for 'policy ethnography' that have come predominantly to the fore as 'advocacy' problems. These problems are seen as ones not only in need of continuous ethical negotiation, but also as fundamentally shaping the ethnographer's self-fashioning as a moral presence in the field (see Singer 1992; Hastrup and Elsass 1990; Browner 1999).[11] As Merrill Singer suggests, 'medical anthropology's reputation as a problem-oriented social science will be decided, in no small measure, by whoever is defining the problems in need of resolution, an issue itself in need of theory-driven examination'. Along with other medical anthropologists, Singer argues that anthropological theory generation has taken second place to the more applied, practical aspects of real-life clinical suffering, and suggests 'the application of theory' (*ibid*:4) might be a feasible way for the future study of local experience. How to develop theory from out of the experiences shaping local moral worlds, as opposed to 'the creation of theory as a bubble-blowing endeavour arrogantly divorced from empirical research', are questions that dovetail precisely with certain concerns currently troubling the medical anthropological study of bioethics.

As the field traditionally concerned with the ethical analysis of scientific and technological developments in Western medicine, mainstream bioethics has subsumed the wide-ranging perspectives of specialists from diverse areas ever since its emergence as a distinct field in the 1960s.[12] While medical ethicists, moral philosophers, lawyers and theologians have found themselves drawn to bioethics debates and thus to the concept of 'value' as forms of cultural reasoning about health and the human life-cycle, medical and social anthropologists have been notably absent from such interdisciplinary endeavour for several rather obvious reasons. Not only has the notion of cultural relativism played little part in the moral thinking of Western bioethics, but anthropology's traditional emphasis on research in non-Western societies also tended to sideline the critical study of developments in Western medicine (Muller 1994; Lieban 1990; Marshall and Koenig 1996).[13]

Further, in seeking to pursue a frame for the comparative study of medical moralities, a growing number of medical anthropologists have questioned the relevance of abstract premises such as the 'four-principles approach' of autonomy, beneficence, nonmaleficence and justice that inform the conventional bioethics rubric.[14] In emphasising the development of 'rational' guidelines for human conduct as codified rules, culture specialists tend to see bioethics as a positivist 'science' of moral absolutes (Muller 1994). Medical anthropologist Arthur Kleinman has been particularly forthright in expounding why these principles may at times present the problem of a dehumanising imposition. Along with other anthropological and non-anthropological commentators, Kleinman attacks the conceptual basis of bioethics, pointing especially to the ethnocentrism inherent in the solipsism of a rights-based view modelled *exclusively* in terms of individual conceptions of the self. Essentially, the gist of such critiques is the place of individualism in cross-cultural approaches to ethics. 'It is not enough to contrast Western and non-Western ethical claims', as he observes, 'since *the very idea of ethics* privileges the

Western view of the individual' (Kleinman 1995:47, emphasis added; cf.
Jacobson-Widding 1997). Given the growth in transnational and capitalist networks of biotechnology, and international health sponsorships more generally, it is surprising to find that (medical) anthropologists have been slow to
take up the theoretical bait of remodelling relations between health, ethics
and human rights. That said, there have been some notable efforts in the
social sciences to broaden, deepen and refine the contours of 'bioethical'
analysis. Pellegrino's (1992) critique for instance on the 'absolutization of
patient autonomy'; Christakis's (1996) revisioning of 'ethical pluralism' in
response to Kleinman's (1995:58) notion of 'deliberative relativism' and
Farmer's (2003) analysis of the 'pathogenic' oversight of medical ethics to treat
inequality as a critical issue in human rights medicine all make important early
advances.

Social anthropologist Wendy James (2000) has also questioned the role and
place of comparative ethnography for the figuring of an alternative analytical framework to conventional biomedical and legally informed approaches to
bioethics. She makes her case in the context of the 'developmental rites' of
Chagga prenatal embryogenesis and childhood growth in order to underscore
the way that 'placing the unborn' requires drawn-out processes of cultural recognition. Opening up questions concerning the legitimacy of pre-life sentience, for
example, James suggests that bioethical 'rights' issues may be re-conceived as
embodied forms of inter-subjective exchange. In this account, the relationship
between ethics and biology is not simply self-evident as, nor indeed reducible to,
the category of 'bioethics'. Rather moral reflection can be built up from the unfamiliar category of well being instantiated as the personhood of maternal-foetal
relations. Here the contributions of anthropology to feminist bioethics promise
to be particularly germane for future conceptualisation of human reproduction and embodiment (see, for example, Donchin and Purdy 1999; Tong 1997;
Wolf 1996).

However, whilst many of these culturally embedded critiques are certainly
suggestive, they have had limited *practical* merit in the specific sense that
medical and social anthropologists clearly have not taken the disciplinary lead
in developing a conceptual and methodological agenda to which bioethicists
would have to respond. This is precisely Paul Farmer's point, as summarised
in his plea for new practices of advocacy, activism and research collaboration
built around 'pragmatic solidarity' (2003:236–41). But there are other reasons
too why anthropologists have been relatively slow to take up the conceptual
bait surrounding bioethics arguments. Relevant here is the legacy of an earlier
generation of social anthropological malaise and its intellectual distancing from
another horizon of 'new science'.

Sociobiology as a new modern synthesis?

When the American entomologist Edward O. Wilson published his book
Sociobiology: The New Synthesis in 1975, its 546 pages provoked extensive
debate and controversy throughout American popular culture. Spawning numerous books, anthologies and lectures and propelled by focused mass media cover-
age, the 'new science' of sociobiology – epitomised particularly by the contents
of Wilson's concluding chapter 'Man: from sociobiology to sociology' – soon
found its way onto the biological curricula of several Ivy-league universities.
The surrounding moral and political debate also galvanised the critical responses
of the Boston-based collective of academics *The Sociobiology Study Group of
Science for the People* and led to various critiques of its racialist implications,
especially through the writing of Stephen Jay Gould and Richard Lewontin.[15]
What exactly was the controversy and why had Wilson's publication sparked
such widespread interest? Though Wilson was hardly the only active propo-
nent of neo-Darwinism at the time – George Price, Bill Hamilton and John
Maynard-Smith in the UK, and Bob Trivers at Harvard had already published
substantially between them – Wilson had effectively identified and formalised
a new field of scientific study. Sociobiology claimed to set out the foundations
of a new science, one that would for the first time provide a biologically based
account of human nature in terms of 'the scientific study of the biological basis
of social behaviour . . . in all kinds of organisms including man' (Wilson 1975:
547). The aim, more specifically, would be to construct and test theories about
the underlying hereditary basis of social behaviour and to promote what Wilson
termed a 'new genetic anthropology'.

Two key responses informed the anthropological rebuttal of sociobiology.
As we shall see, this critique remained limited in scope and for several reasons
attracted only a small number of social and cultural anthropologists, notably
Marshall Sahlins, Ashley Montagu, Edmund Leach, Derek Freeman and Marvin
Harris. First and foremost, anthropologists criticised the 'biologism' (Montagu
1980:5) and reductionism inherent in sociobiological explanations of human
behaviour. Montagu, Freeman and Leach all conceded that a good deal of human
social behaviour may well have a genetic basis, but they also insisted that it is
a very different proposition to claim that such behaviour is itself genetically
determined. In short, the anthropologists thought that Wilson had simply paid
lip service to the complexity that characterised the interaction between genes
and the environment. As against a view stressing the determinative or deci-
sive actions of the genes, anthropologists unanimously countered with a view
of the constitutive forces of culture as the human-made, self-fashioning part
of the environment. Second and related to this, these social commentators all

took exception to the assimilation of anthropology into the epistemological pretensions of 'unity' that Wilson had outlined as the future of the so-called 'Modern Synthesis'. In outlining what can be seen as the epistemological pretensions of a 'new' modern synthesis, Wilson boldly proclaimed that 'the humanities and social sciences shrink to specialised branches of biology' (1975:547). Further, he held that one of the functions of sociobiology was 'to reformulate the foundations of the social sciences' so that they became 'truly biologized', and anthropology (together with sociobiology) constitutes 'the sociobiology of a single species' (*ibid*:574). Wilson went on to develop these ideas outlining in a couple of subsequent articles why sociobiology represents a privileged way of knowing over and beyond the social sciences and the humanities. 'The role of sociobiology with reference to human beings, then, is to place the social sciences within a biological framework, a framework constructed from a synthesis of evolutionary studies, genetics, population biology, ecology, animal behaviour, psychology and anthropology' (Wilson 1976:342).

Though Wilson himself wonders 'whether the social sciences can be truly biologicised in this fashion' (1975:4), the vision appears to be articulated in terms of unequivocal pretensions to disciplinary hegemony. With the claim that biology represents the 'antidiscipline' of the social sciences, Wilson made a simultaneous move to suggest that anthropology, in particular 'has already become *the social science closest to sociobiology*' (Wilson 1977:134, emphasis added). Since the task of an antidiscipline within a scientific hierarchy was to reduce explanations in a 'higher' field to explanations in the field immediately 'beneath', it thus fell to sociobiology – as the 'antidiciscipline' of anthropology – to demonstrate that the explanation of cultural practices was actually fathomable from biological processes themselves! One might, of course, be prompted to invert such hierarchical rankings of synthetic union into a more modest reckoning and say that those sciences relating specifically to humans could best be placed – through not necessarily subsumed – within an anthropological framework. Ashley Montagu (1980:6) had already proposed such a possibility, though in very general terms. What seems to be the curious point, and indeed curiously missing from subsequent 'postmodernist' commentary, is why these critical remarks should have remained such a singular, uncontested and uncanonised voice within the profession at large.

The vulgarity of sociobiology

Marshall Sahlins (1976) was the first anthropologist to formulate an extended review and critique of the new biological science. *The Use and Abuse of Biology* assimilates in fairly cursory style a range of material from the existing ethnographic record so as to illustrate how the sociobiological focus on animal behaviour as a template for human action completely overlooked the significance of cultural forms of social organisation and belief. Sociobiology was, Sahlins argued, a 'vulgar' science that borrowed stealthily from culture by transposing anthropomorphic tendencies to animal behaviour and then passing off these same tendencies as 'natural'. The view that there is nothing in society that was not first evident in non-human organisms, and that there exists in nature a fixed correspondence between innate human drives, social behaviour and social institutions were seen as deeply damaging forms of vulgar reductionism. From an anthropological viewpoint, to suggest that violence and warfare between men arise from an innate male disposition to aggression simply sullied the cultural context of human interaction, social exchange and sociality. 'Between "aggression" and Vietnam, "sexuality" and cross-cousin marriage, "reciprocal altruism" and the exchange of red shell necklaces, biology offers us merely an enormous intellectual void. Within the void left by biology lies the whole of anthropology' (Sahlins 1977:16).

Sahlins set about reclaiming culture with his critique of 'kin selection' that aimed to show how people invent kinship as a social form. We will see later how local kinship practices in the context of cultures of predisposition and predictive genetic testing technology carry forward Sahlins' disdain for the sociobiological claim that 'knowledge of genealogical relationships is always the secret wisdom of the genes' (Sahlins 1977:23). For the moment, let me simply draw out how Sahlins' analysis unfolds as a critical historiography of the notion of evolution and the related ideology and idiom of 'natural selection'.

According to Sahlins, natural selection is intimately bound up with the rise of late capitalism in Western Euro-American culture. The optimisation thesis of gene-selectionist approach, or what Sahlins calls the 'self-maximisation of the individual genotype' (1977:4) is both a literal and metaphorical rendition of the sociobiological belief that the inclusive fitness of individual selection stands for 'an economic metaphor of enterprising individualism' (1977:20). Macpherson's (1962) thesis of 'possessive individualism' thus transmutes here into a form of 'genetic capitalism' (Sahlins 1977:72) and accounts for social exploitation in terms of the causal factors of economic domination. In this materialist reading, the sociobiological preoccupation with nature-culture co-evolution (see especially Lumsden and Wilson 1981) is analysed in terms of a specific dialectical interaction: the natural difference between groups of non-human organisms stands also for the means to explain – as cultural event – the social inequalities experienced by different people. Sahlins phrases this famously as 'an endless reciprocal exchange between social Darwinism and natural capitalism' (1977:xv) that takes formative shape as 'the culturalisation of nature and the naturalisation of culture' (1977:105).

'Culturgens' and 'exogenetic' culture

Derek Freeman (1980) on the other hand engages this dialectic somewhat differently insisting on a 'dual track' pathway of genetic and cultural evolution, the latter representing a second and superimposed layer upon the pre-existing system of genetic change. I don't want to focus here on why Freeman should have come to this position, nor why he elaborated his ensuing critique of 'geneticism' (1980:213) in terms that first addressed the contrasting behaviour systems of the 'closed' (non-adaptive responses) of the mosquito and the 'open' (culturally adaptive) responses of the Japanese macaque. What I do want to bring home is Freeman's insistence on 'exogenetic culture' (1980:205, 206, 209) as the social inheritance and inter-generational transmission of [exogenetic] information as choices made by human agents throughout the course of history. What matters in Freeman's account, and indeed runs through the entirety of this book as a central concern, is how people act to convert inherited [genetic] 'instructions' into sources of social information, or indeed, misinformation. The worthwhile point then – so far as Freeman's analysis is concerned – is that we already have here the intimations of how the agentic processes of so-called 'exogenetic information' (1980:206) contrast fundamentally with the gene's eye view of natural selection as a 'blind decision-making process' (Wilson 1978:197) As just stated, this is a view I develop in considerable detail in the second part of this book, particularly as I trace how various kin affected by Huntington's are implicated in the knowledge flows that constitute the information-exchange processes of predictive genetics.

Now, whilst Freeman formulated his critique through the redeeming features of 'exogenetic culture', Edmund Leach was busy attacking the sociobiological concept of 'culturgens'. 'The proper study of mankind' is the title of one of Leach's (1978) damning reviews.[16] Like Sahlins, Leach had been motivated to respond critically to the claims of the new science, and just after the publication of Sahlins' *Use and Abuse* he took up the anthropological bait, not – it seems – without a dash of sceptical amusement. Commenting on Wilson's (1978) latest book entitled *On Human Nature*, Leach observes wryly that 'my personal reaction is boredom rather than hostility' (1978:x). He proceeded to admonish the text for its rambling lexicon, self-contradictory and unoriginal comments, and worst of all, its grossly misinformed handling of ethnographic data. A couple of years later Wilson (1981) proposed the co-evolutionary model of 'culturgens' in his next major treatise. This was entitled *Genes, Mind and Culture*, and was co-written with the physicist Charles Lumsden. When Leach (1981) wrote up his review of this in the science journal *Nature*, laconic amusement had turned into the more acerbic tone of wondrous bemusement. 'This book comes so close to being a parody of the genre to which it belongs', Leach wrote 'that I have difficulty in believing it is not intended as an academic hoax' (1981:267).

One might see in retrospect how Leach's doubts about the intellectual authenticity of sociobiology and the related pretensions of the 'Modern Synthesis' surface as an early manifestation of postmodernist critique. To a certain extent, Leach appears – at least in an internal sense for anthropology – as a visionary forerunner of the 1990s Science Wars: he had given voice to much of what was to provoke the scandal of the Sokal hoax-affair (see above '"hot" science, "cold" ethics?'). But what specifically was the substance of Leach's 'prophetic' objection?

Leach basically argued that Lumsden and Wilson's examples of 'gene-culture translation' were wholly amiss. Having dipped cavalierly into certain ethnographic literature, Lumsden and Wilson had sought to demonstrate the existence of 'chains of causation' (Leach's term) that link 'principal culturgens' with 'derivative culturgens' as certain epigenetic rules. As Leach remarks, it is not even clear how the authors want to mobilise genetics with their erroneous suggestion that patrilineal, patrilocal and polygnous forms of social organisation always preclude female initiation rites, for example. The clitoridectomy practices prevalent amongst East African nomadic pastoralists have nothing obviously to do with sociobiological genetics, and in any case, Lumsden and Wilson were clearly lacking in their knowledge of the indigenous marriage rules prevalent in different cultures. By equating the concept of 'culturgens' with readily identifiable entities, as though it were possible simply to equate the whole of 'culture' with clusters of given traits, sociobiologists were seen to be guilty of mobilising the concept of culture in a way anthropologists could not recognise and certainly could not accept. In Wilson and Lumsden's hands, 'culture' had turned into an over-homogenised synthesis of 'custom' that was simply subsumed within the 'phoney mathematical apparatus' (Leach 1981:268) of numerous diagrams, graphs and sophisticated-looking algebraic equations. In this 'synthetic' account, the non-anthropological treatment of culture amounted to little more than a crude statistical treatment of human behaviour, all of which prompted Leach to conclude that 'the jargon loaded take-over bid proposed by Lumsden and Wilson is just bunk' (1981:267).

Commentary and summary

A quarter of a century ago, a handful of anthropological critiques of sociobiology – as well as other social science-related commentary – reviewed some
of the problems with the central tenets of neo-Darwinian evolutionary biology.
These anthropological critiques highlighted the key omission of considerations
of 'culture', in particular the ethnocentrism underpinning the notions of 'natural
selection', 'inclusive fitness' and 'kin selection', however they did not go on
to explore the cultural implications of the genetics of sociobiology beyond its
potential disciplinary encroachment of anthropology itself. Of course, from a
conventional anthropological perspective that took as its own basic unit of study
the cultural beliefs and practices of small-scale, non-industrialised non-Western
societies, sociobiology was not a set of beliefs that was likely to impact directly
on the discipline's core theoretical orientation of the time.

Now whether or not one subscribes to the various permutations of cultural
materialism, Marvin Harris's cautions appear particularly suggestive and forward for the time. Asking rhetorically 'who is to blame for sociobiology', and
probing why it was that the sociobiologists could at least appear to advance
their 'modern synthesis' across anthropological terrain (and other humanities),
he identifies the underdevelopment of anthropological theory as 'an intellectual
disaster area' (Harris 1980:333). On this count, witness how Sahlins is at pains
to justify and explain the 'new' interventions of an American anthropologist
into 'familiar' cultural ground: 'Now if the natives concerned were of some
other tribe, the anthropologist would without hesitation think it his task to try
to discover that relation. Yet if there is culture anywhere in humanity, there is
culture even in America, and no less obligation on the anthropologist's part to
consider it as such, though he finds it even more difficult to work as an observing
participant than as a participant observer. I should like to treat the ideological
issues in this kind of ethnographic spirit' (Sahlins 1977:xiii). Certainly in the
1970s, ideas about the hereditary transmission of physical substance so obviously concerned the origins myths of Western societies that the specifically
cultural study of genetics as a 'native' science held little sustained conceptual
interest, and was thus precluded from entering the mainstream as a systematic
programme of anthropological research. The point to note is that this omission
parallels the way medical anthropologists, up until very recently, neglected the
field of biomedicine and bioethics as a mainstream preoccupation of medical
anthropology (see above 'anthropology, ethics and bioethics').

Insofar as these anthropological critiques in the 1970s did potentially pave the
way for the substantive reconfiguration of biology in specifically cultural terms,
it is possible to see – again in retrospect – how these critical comments remained

distinctively peripheral to the future *theoretical* development of Anglophone socio-cultural anthropology. This is not to downplay the important work reflecting the anthropological turn to questions of subjectivity, 'the body' and gender-related issues from the mid-1980s onwards, but rather to note that the cultural study of human genetics *per se* did not become a substantive part of that post-modernist agenda, nor indeed of any other theoretical agenda. If thirty years ago structuralist-inspired anthropologists generally could not see how a focus on the study of the origins of culture should include centrally in its theoretical remit what was quite obviously the ethnocentrism of certain Western scientific biologists, we need to ask how much has actually changed today. Judging by current-day anthropological curricula, the study of the links between culture and human genetics, and (say) the cultural relevance of the ideology of genetic behaviourism for populations, are not seen as serious *core* theoretical issues for undergraduates and postgraduates in most British universities. In fact, the subject of genetics happens to be taken much more seriously by just about everybody else! It is 'colonised' from all sorts of directions: from ethicists, lawyers, sociologists, political theorists and philosophers to visual artists, communication technicians, public education specialists and, of course, scientists! More notably still, many of these non-anthropological voices claim to be talking about the relationship between culture and genetics, occupying ostensibly the very ground of critical anthropological investigation (see, for example, Clarke and Parsons 1997).

Yet besides the problem of ethnocentrism, there were other obvious shortcomings making the claims of sociobiological theory superfluous to mainstream socio-cultural anthropology. 'The blind decision-making process of natural selection' (Wilson 1978:197), bolstered in turn by the 'gene's eye' pretensions of Dawkinsian sociobiology elaborated in such texts as *The Selfish Gene* (1976) and *The Blind Watchmaker* (1987) was clearly not the stuff of local sentience and indigenous perception. Though sociobiology was about the biological basis of mankind's behaviour and concerned the natural evolution of the animal and human species – and the ostensible evolutionary links between the two – actually there were quite obviously no living people in these accounts! It became inconceivable for socio-cultural anthropologists – as opposed to biophysical anthropologists such as Lionel Tiger, Robin Fox, Napoleon Chagnon, Bill Irons and other anthropologists working in conjunction with early evolutionary psychologists such as John Tooby and Lena Cosmides at Harvard – to imagine how they could make sustained *ethnographic* inroads into the fetishised object known as 'the gene'. True, David Schneider's work on the cultural symbols of natural substance took up folk concepts of heredity as part of a conceptual critique of North American kinship forms. The point though was that it was technically and methodologically difficult for anthropologists then to come to grips ethnographically with the space of interiorised genes. It was difficult in the sense of formulating feasible research topics that would be recognisable as a specific locale to which a fieldworker could go and watch things unfold over time. Evolutionary biology simply did not lend itself to critical anthropological sensibilities, nor importantly did it yoke well with conventional ethnographic methodology.

Furthermore it is all too possible that anthropology's own professional structuration of symbolic prestige, for instance the professional requirements of the discipline for extended ethnographic immersion, inhibited the systematic development of the cultural study of biology as a form of legitimate anthropological critique. In this vein, it is important to recognise that those few cultural anthropologists who did bother to engage themselves directly with the new sociobiology were writing in a theoretical and philosophical style about the biosciences as a *theory* of human biology and human culture. This, then, was cultural anthropology at work through the devices of critical juxtaposition and the inchoate 'playing off' of one set of theoretical beliefs about culture – drawn in the main from the existing ethnographic record – against another set of non-anthropological beliefs. It was not so much that sociobiology represented a 'strange' sub-set of otherwise 'familiar' Western beliefs, but rather that a handful of anthropologists were moved to defend the territory of 'culture' from what was then seen as unwarranted disciplinary encroachment. Hence in response to Lumsden and Wilson's (1981) notion of 'culturgens', we have, for example, Leach's (1981) admonition of the symbolic violence of rape, itself an intellectual precursor of the 'Science Wars', and Freeman's 'exogenetic' rebuttal of sociobiology as the 'antidiscipline' of anthropology.

Yet it is not until the end of the century, and a good few decades since the advent of sociobiology, that cultural historians and other social theorists effectively rethink the idiom of 'culturgens' as convoluted processes of gene-culture 'mistranslation'. The following section briefly reviews how recent turn-of-the-century social critiques outside the field of anthropology carry forward in significant ways the earlier anthropological critiques of genetic reductionism, as outlined above. I restrict myself to certain aspects of the importation of the cybersciences into mid-century biology, outlining only certain aspects I see as constructive critical pointers for a revised 'postgenomic' synthesis between culture-and-genetics. In particular, by examining critiques that have deconstructed how the informational idiom of DNA became a universal quasi-language, we shall see how Freeman's concern with 'exogenetic' information, as well as the general anthropological concern with language as one of the key indices of 'humanness', is given a firmer and sharper cultural twist. Up to a point.

Code words

When James Watson and Francis Crick claimed in 1953 to have discovered the biochemical structure of DNA as the coiled conformation of two complementary and anti-parallel chains, their visualisation of the 'double helix' as a continuous sequence of spiralling information was also a moment of cultural recognition. The human body, it was claimed, comprised a universally encoded language whose 'grammar' shapes the kind of person we each become, and informs the quintessential metabolic exchanges of virtually every organism one cares to examine. According to this view, the interiorised corporeal arrangement of the molecular substances known as adenine, cytosine, guanine and thymine reveals a 'language of the genes', or more tellingly still, encompasses what scientists have named the 'book of life'.[17] It is not simply noteworthy that Western trained molecular biologists, clinical and research geneticists all seem to talk in terms of a formal syntax made up from the key referents of 'code', 'message', 'messenger', 'instructions' and 'blueprint', but that several secondary analyses have borrowed so freely these 'language of life' analogies. Literally reworking the book of life idiom, Matt Ridley (1999) even goes so far as to re-present the human genome as the *autobiography* of a species in twenty-three chapters. The geneticist Steve Jones calls his overview (1993) of biology, history and the evolutionary future *The Language of the Genes*, and Daniel Kevles and Leroy Hood's (1992) otherwise critical exploration of the social implications of the Human Genome Project similarly falls under the titular rubric of *The Code of Codes*. It is the readiness then with which social value has been imputed to these biological facts, rather than the constellation of these helix-like sequences themselves, that finally make these biological chains into links that can interconnect. Or perhaps snap. For it is not the case that biological chains of nucleotides are the only way of isolating sequences of DNA as meaningful 'secrets of life'.

Critical scholarship in recent years by cultural historians of science and feminist philosophers of biology has sought to challenge mainstream scientific and popular representations of the genetic code. Much of this work, in its exploration of the relationship between cultural norms, metaphor and technical development, considers the performative effects of language in biology and may best be viewed as one arm of an emergent critical social theory of human genetic science.[18] Perhaps one of the most suggestive insights of this body of literature is the speculation that early American geneticists went ahead and attributed

agency to the gene simply on account of their own partial and incomplete understanding of complex biochemical processes. Evelyn Fox Keller (1995) argues
that the scientists' penchant for gene action and internal agency simply helped
to 'cover up' – or divert attention away from – inadequate science. In brief,
the problem for geneticists was that they could not proffer verifiable evidence
concerning the grounds whereby ontological essence could be attributed to the
gene (see Fox Keller 1995:10). According to this reading, genetics has always
been a partial and inchoate local theory about the biological origins of human
life.

Lily Kay carries such insights further in her comprehensive account of the
cultural history of the genetic code in mid-twentieth century genetic science,
Who Wrote the Book of Life? Documenting the key paradigm shift of protein synthesis that accompanied Watson and Crick's breakthrough and examining the
race to determine 'code words' between different genetic teams and laboratories
in the 1960s as a prophetic harbinger of the 1980s transnational Human Genome
Project, this analysis contends that the genetic code, as informational and scriptural representations of heredity, became naturalised as a basic fact of life and
authorless form of 'genomic textuality' (2000:331). Though Kay's account predates the articulations of the 'Modern Synthesis', this detailed archival research
takes the anthropological theoretical critique of sociobiology one step further
by showing how concepts of hereditary substance came to be reconfigured by
genetic science as predominantly informational. Crucially, the field of biology
was reconfigured as the re-description of physical and biological phenomena in
terms of the then dominant post-war models of information theory and cyber-
netics. Heredity was seen as isomorphic with a programmed communication
system that was governed by a code and that transferred 'linguistic information'
through the cell and cycles of life. Molecules and organisms were seen as texts
and as systems of information storage and transfer. Adapting Norbert Wiener's
version of 'molecular biosemiotics', Kay refers to this as 'the new biosemiotics
of communication' (2000:xviii). At the same time, in displacing the concept
of specificity that had informed the pre-genetic protein view of life, the informational idiom as applied to biology became 'a metaphor of a metaphor, a
catachresis, and a signifier without a referent' (2000:24). Essentially the icon-
oclastic imagery of code breaking depended on an illusory rhetoric. Even the
most powerful computerised technologies could not really *break* the genetic
code because technically speaking – from linguistic and cryptanalytic perspectives – the genetic code is no more a real code than DNA is a natural language.
Comprised solely of three-letter words, 'DNA linguistics' lacks, *inter alia*,
phonemic features, semantics, punctuation marks, and intersymbol restrictions.
It is, as Kay rightly observes, a powerful metaphor for the correlations between

nucleic and amino acids, and an historically specific and culturally contingent imaginary 'period piece' – a manifestation and legacy of the post cold-war information age.

By exposing the hollowness of the claim that heredity represents a kind of 'information processing' and the related belief that the genome is a sort of computer, Kay's analysis further opens up the gap between biological and cultural processes of information reckoning. By identifying this gap, and showing why it is so significant, the question about legitimate cultural authorship encapsulated by the book's very title exposes another salient issue: namely how genetic information can be converted into knowledge as processes of social value construction. In addition, by showing how scriptural technology was poised as the interface of several interlocking postwar discourses such as physics, mathematics, information theory, cryptanalysis, electronic computing and linguistics, Kay highlights how there was nothing inevitable about the mid-century uptake of informational idiom. The crucial point is that there could always be other ways of knowing and accessing what counts as knowledge. Fifty years ago, the interactionist properties of the information metaphor provided the potential to traffic analogies between different areas of Western science.[19] Simply put, this metaphorisation of information worked as an interdisciplinary and cultural medium of exchange, yet curiously, the importation into biology of analogical modes of reasoning was not theorised as the culturalisation of biology. In reneging the advances of the 'Modern Synthesis', the earlier anthropological critiques of sociobiology did not follow up how 'information' itself could be re-theorised in extra-scientific terms as the rematerialisation of biology. Though an important clue had been laid by the metaphorical power of the informational idiom, the gap between biological and cultural processes of information exchange as ways of knowing, did not become a centrepiece of these 1970s anthropological critiques.

Summary

In switching perspective from macro-evolutionary processes to the continuous chain of signification that shapes nucleotide sequences, the field of biology is opened up for critical study in terms of its metaphorical value for the scientific construction of 'man'. In so doing, Kay's analysis illuminates how the dominant discourse of 'gene action' that framed mid-twentieth century molecular biology exposes the Western reification of genes as *the* basis of all life.

Narrating the New Predictive Genetics considers the question of the cultural rematerialisation and metaphorisation of biology in terms that further challenge the scientific hegemony of genetic information. What I want to discuss, as part of a broader project questioning the feasibility of a 'postgenomic' synthesis, is the active importation of cultural analogies and metaphors as anthropological forms of reasoning into Western science. In brief, my argument is that certain metaphorical fields in genetics have been occluded from critical and reflexive consideration due to the heavy semantic emphasis that scientists and non-scientists have placed, and indeed continue to place, on the informational idiom. Further, in societies where genetics now has become one of the central idioms through which folk theories of human origins and cultural development can be expressed and publicly validated, the active importation of culture into biology is seen to justify ethical attributions and analyses.[20] Nowhere is this explicitness made more explicit a social convention than with the recent discursive appeals to the enterprise of 'genethics'. But as technology literally remodels man [*sic*] along a continuum of moral debate and consensus, the place of ethical inventiveness depends on thinking how to re-theorise the 'proper' study of mankind (cf. Leach 1978).[21]

A genethics synthesis for the 21st century?

Genethics

Like many of the technologies it describes, genethics is a 'recombinant' term derived from the hybrid compound of the spliced word 'genetics' (genetics/ethics). Taking as its object of study the health-related gene technologies emanating from genome research, it denotes a narrower and more precise delimitation of the field of bioethics. Usually this is seen to encompass a growing number of present and hypothetical scenarios some of which bridge procreative and genetic science, or so-called 'reprogenics'. Genethics practitioners may be debating anything ranging from stem cell therapy and the immortalisation of cell lines, therapeutic cloning, modification of the germ-line, transgenic experimental therapies and the creation of genetically modified organisms, to name just a few concerns.

Much of the existing literature relating to genethics is broad, often prescriptive in substance and interdisciplinary in its remit. From the perspective of public international law and international health agencies, the work of UNESCO (United Nations Educational and Scientific Cultural Organisation), the WHO (World Health Organisation) and the CIOMS (Council for International Organisations of Medical Sciences) has been directed towards establishing international ethical norms and standards for genetic testing technologies (see Bankowski and Capron 1990). Concurrent with the development of international instruments and relevant directives in biomedicine (see above pp. 29–31) a number of geneticists have also turned their hand to the medium of popular science writing. In an attempt to reach the sensibilities of a wider audience, a new breed of genetic philosophers make suggestive interventions concerning guidelines for 'genetic responsibility' (e.g. Suzuki and Knudtson 1990). A more self-consciously proactive strand of genetic activists is also emerging, often grouped around science policy communication, consumer and campaigning organisations, united by concerns about runaway technologies, gene patenting and the future of genome developmental progress. Tokar's (2001) detailed volume on indigenous and local responses to global genomics has a section devoted to medical genetics, science and human rights with contributors ranging from indigenous grass-roots health campaigners to those with conventional science backgrounds, academic sociologists, ethicists and life science policy experts. Note however that despite the volume's explicitly global focus, the reader will find no indexed entry or cross-references for, say, the terms 'culture', 'anthropology' or 'ethnography'. Where Stephen Jay Gould could cross over into the domain he named as 'the anthropology of morals', the current genethics literature tends simply to bypass the question of what it is that makes the explicitly cultural contribution to these debates important, distinctive and timely. Again there are exceptions. Suzuki and Knudtson's (1990) formulation of nine 'genethic principles' is about as far away from an anthropological analysis as one could get. However, the authors – a geneticist and freelance science writer respectively – are unusual in one thing. Right at the end of their analysis, explicit reference is made to the potential value of insights from cultural anthropology. How, they ask, can anthropologists contribute to the formulation of new 'moral maps'? How can anthropology specifically help to 'forge a new, cross-cultural synthesis of moral values that address the most disturbing questions raised by modern molecular genetics and genetic engineering?' (1990:338)

Philosopher David Heyd (1994:23) suggests that genethics may be seen as 'ways of worldmaking' and that techno-genesis problems may best be considered beyond the conceptual boundaries of a normative ethics. Heyd's work takes a more philosophical angle than Suzuki and Knudtson and attempts to limit the field of genethics to the specific issues arising from the creation of unborn *potential* persons. Like others, he considers possible ethical baselines for the moral conceptualisation of the being and well being of 'pre-human' persons who are, by definition, themselves incapable of moral discrimination. This suggests the conceptual problem of how to think a viable morality outside of the philosophical framework of sovereign autonomy. With their keen sense of an individual and conscious self, such questioning for Euro-Americans may be seen as a tantalising 'experimental' moment. Genethics as practice and critical theoretical discourse puts into centre-view the intriguing possibility that the category of the moral person may in fact be founded, at least in part, upon a non-knowing pre-subject. This 'person' may be exemplified and made manifest culturally as genetic information that others have about various extracted human body parts, tissues, organs or DNA.

It is at this point that an anthropological approach and social critique of 'genethics' may find some purpose and justification. Not only can social anthropology lay claim to an established record of comparative research on the diverse practices surrounding 'coming into being', it has sought also to expound the variable meanings attributed to local concepts of personhood and kinship as indigenous theories of gestation, birth and fertility. Indeed, it is partly for this reason that anthropological interest in the new reproductive technologies since the late 1980s began to question the impact of 'assisted' forms of conception for notions of nature and the generativity of social relations.[22] In the event, speculation about the medicalisation of kinship has opened up a significant set of research questions about the relationship between procreative technology and previously unexplored 'facts' about personhood. At much the same time and aside from developments relating to Western science and technology, a number of social anthropologists have questioned how indigenous conceptions of morality – as cultural attributions of value – might be expressed as local conceptions of the 'self'. As opposed to early prescriptive definitions of morality engendered by social wholes and disembodied beings, ethnographic work since the 1970s has pointed to the significance of emotional and moral knowledge for constructs of the self,[23] and some of this work has taken a specific health inflection.[24] Anthropologists have also become increasingly interested in approaching concepts of personhood in terms of the connection between moral relations and the negotiation of forms of 'indeterminate ambiguity' (see e.g. Evens 1982; Jackson 1982; Shore 1990; Beidelman 1993).

And yet despite these parallel avenues into questions of morality and forms of 'uncertain' personhood, anthropology and genethics have not engaged in *active* dialogue with each other. Generally, anthropology has tended not to present itself explicitly to genethicists. This is to say it has not been usual practice for anthropologists interested in the new biotechnology to take their findings back *directly* to the bioethics forum, either as critical constructive engagement or, recalling Parkin's and Pocock's earlier plea, as development of theory generation in this area. The two literatures thus have remained largely separate repositories of knowledge about how to think through and engage with morality-in-action. Let me offer at this juncture an example of an alternative 'way in'.

Crossing continents, crossing chromosomes

It has been said that the new genetic maps of the Human Genome Project parallel, if not exceed in cultural value, the maps of discovery made by the voyagers of the New World. Traversing new geophysical territory and forging new medico-scientific representations of human bodies – evidently these are separate exploratory journeys that utilise different material technologies of conquest even if both have relied on a cartographic imagery of frontiers, progress, habitation and occupation.[25] However when the physical space of the body itself comes to be literalised as a new expansive territory and medium for objectification, how does yesterday's sea-faring or plantation slave join hands with today's victims of global bio-piracy, genetic commodification and the mercantile trading of body parts for profit?

The question of who 'owns' the human genome and what kind of knowledge is engendered by such biological resources was a fundamental part of both the science and ethics surrounding the 'breakthrough' of the first so-called 'rough draft' of the sequenced human genome. The International Human Genome Sequencing Consortium, representing the collaborative effort of twenty laboratories and hundreds of scientists from around the world, declared itself a public research project from the outset and made its collections of sequence data available to all those connected to the Internet.[26] At the same time as the Consortium completed its results in early 2001, Celera Genomics, a privately owned US company, published a 'rival' draft sequence with slightly different data. Headed at the time by Craig Venter, a genetics entrepreneur intent on selling the sequence information to pharmaceutical companies, Celera decided not to make its data freely accessible. Many science activists and researchers subsequently condemned the company's findings as an example of unethical science (see The International Human Genome Mapping Consortium 2001 and Venter *et al.* 2001). Now stepping back momentarily from these ownership controversies, the social scientist might profitably look again at how molecular biology makes its own body of knowledge. When genetic scientists are recognised primarily as parallel voyagers traversing a microcosmos of corporeal movement, exchange and unpredictable bodily transfer, how are former nature-culture dichotomies reconfigured as value in a regime of 'biosociality'? (Rabinow 1992). How is biology rewritten as ethical landscape?

Despite the fact that social anthropology and molecular genetics are both relatively young intellectual traditions whose disciplinary credentials originate from around the turn of the last century, each now extends across diverse sub-disciplinary fields. Each discipline also has produced a voluminous literature of methods, models and conceptual refinement. For its part, social anthropology

first became recognised as a formal 'science' of society and of man ('anthro-
pos') with the professional transition to ethnographic field methods initiated by
Bronislaw Malinowski during and immediately after the First World War years.
Genetics in the early 1900s had formalised the laws of Mendelian inheritance
by incorporating insights about the recurrent traits of cross-bred peas into cell
biology and was set to make advances in chromosome analysis and the development of model organisms. Not only are these subject concerns conceptually,
philosophically and methodologically diverse, they also represent seemingly
disparate disciplinary fields with little obvious reason or occasion for sustained
encounter or cross-dialogue.

For the non-scientist 'visiting' for the first time the syntax of classical Western genetics, and especially for the interested anthropologist watchful of the
practices of gene-based technology and its applications, there is however a
certain irony to this mutually enforced avoidance of the disciplinary 'other'
as cross-relation. Those with anthropological sensibilities may even delight in
finding a rich imagery of indigenous anatomy whose linkages can be probed first
in terms of the kinds of connections geneticists imagine they make as they take
apart the constituent elements of the human or non-human cell, analyse protein
structures and enzyme conversions. The second possible delight comes in seeing how such microcosmic endeavours of cell analysis themselves comprise a
metonymic rendition of ordered creation and universe constellation. Genetics,
in this sense, has always been a partial and inchoate local story (or scientific
'theory') about the biological origins of human life, and no matter whether or
not one believes in this origins story *in toto*, it is the idioms that scientists deploy
to tell their account that fascinate. In turn, geneticists might find it refreshing
to consider how certain of their indigenous expressions carry an unexpected
anthropological resonance. But first a few words on spatial arrangements.

Of particular interest is the way that genes have been conceptualised by scientists as the interiorised parts of bodily persons or animal models. In humans,
these parts are said to occupy certain positions within a spatialised cosmology that is the human body.[27] Genes and alleles (variant forms of a gene) are
said to have 'loci' and are known by way of certain spatial 'markers' that are
identified along string-like structures called chromosomes. Each gene, in other
words, occupies a specific place, or locus, on one particular chromosome and
is simultaneously part of a sequence of linearly arranged substances known
bio-chemically as nucleotides. Genes, in other words, are identified as locations whose whereabouts, surmised through 'linkage analysis' and the attempt
to plot gene transfers during cell division at fertilisation, may be further sys-
temised through 'mapping' resources, many of which have been developed
through recent work on the Human Genome Initiative.[28]

Open just about any introductory genetics textbook and you will soon see these are replete with descriptions about how chromosomes *move* and cross-over during cell division. Accounts of 'meiosis' describing the process of cell division and the formation of the egg and sperm cells at fertilisation are indeed the classic staple of every genetics curricula. Crossing over takes place when a stretch of one chromosome changes place with a segment of its corresponding (homologous) chromosome. Cell division therefore is a complex and elaborate staging of positions, a particular cosmological world of shifting transformation and *chiasma* (indigenous term) involving place, movement, crossing, splitting, exchange, transfer and the linkage of divergent chromosomal parts.[29] The classical genetics texts tell us that chromosomes at different stages of meiotic division 'come together and lie alongside each other' (at the zygotene and pachytene stage). Chromatids are said to 'exchange sequences by crossing-over' (pachytene stage and chiasma). Homologous pairs of chromosomes are said to 'orient and align themselves along the equator of the spindle' (metaphase 1 and 2) or 'to move towards opposite poles of the spindle (anaphase 1 and 2).[30] As the composite assemblages of a variety of markers ('places'), genes are therefore entities that move about within and between persons[31], though these intra and cross-regional transfers do not always shape up in ways you would necessarily like or expect. A misplaced or lost gene may entail what is called an 'interstitial deletion' or an unexpected 'recombination event'. As an expression of non-linkage this may mean you are born with a congenital disease or may suffer in later years from a so-called 'inherited' condition. Interestingly for anthropology, the science of genetics attempts to understand the biochemical mechanisms of heredity in terms of a spatialised methodology of regional mapping and comparative distantiation.[32] When geneticists attempt to measure the frequencies of so-called recombination events (arrangements at meiosis) between any two genes, what they are interested in conceptualising is the proximity of the physical distance between these biological entities. The name that they give to both the method of tracking the frequency of recombination, as well as to the object of recombination itself, is the term 'linkage map'.

Arguably though the crowning metaphor underpinning the spatialised methodology of genetic knowledge is that of 'translocation'. The genetic concept of translocation directly captures the anthropological imagination because in the very moment of movement that is chromosomal exchange and gamete transformation, it engages a particular notion of value – namely, the chance of imperfection. As an imagery of life-in-the-making, translocation is the story of the organism's recombination, but more than that, it is the story of coming into being as essential fallibility. It is about beginning from a position of recognised displacement.

Geneticists routinely refer to the technical term translocation to describe what happens when a fragment of one chromosome sporadically and accidentally breaks off and becomes attached to a different chromosome, either in a somatic cell or while a gamete is being made during fertilisation (meiosis).[33] There are many ways in which so-called 'accidents' at meiosis can result in chromosome rearrangements, duplications and deletions, some of which are consequential for the health of future offspring, and others (implicating only carrier status, for example) that are assumed relatively innocuous. Now, classical genetics looks as though it has plundered the best of anthropological gift theory when it goes on to identify a 'reciprocal translocation' as 'an exchange of segments between two different (non-homologous) chromosomes that form reattachments in new combinations' (Sudbery 1998:18; Mange and Mange 1999:291–2). Admittedly, there is no explicit reference here to the significance of temporal deferral as Mauss (1990) originally identified, so we can at least see that the workings of reciprocity are not governed in these particular exchanges by the intentions of moral and socially invested cultural agents. Genetics concentrates instead on spatialisation and the technicalities of proximity as degrees of disembodied pathology. A 'Robertsonian translocation' refers, for example, to translocations between and among acrocentric chromosomes (i.e. numbers 13, 14, 15, 21 and 22) that join near their centomeres (the point at which the two arms of a chromosome join together end to end) to form a single new chromosome. So-called balanced translocations (in which loss of chromosome material on the short arms results in no phenotypical change) are contrasted with 'unbalanced translocations' signifying non-reciprocal exchange of a chromosome segment (namely, when a pair of translocated chromosomes are not inherited together in a gamete).[34] We thus can see that the idiom of translocation evokes a combined imagery and complex of associations whose value turns on the disembodied impetus of: (1) [being in] place; (2) [being in] movement; and (3) [being as] error. When geneticists refer to the term translocation to describe chromosome breakage across biological space, they are clearly conceptualising the event of translocation in terms of the particular form of life thereby arising (balanced and viable or unbalanced and unviable). They are not, unlike approaches from the social sciences and humanities, drawing upon conceptions of physical distance to think about how processes and identities unfold over time as embodied knowledge and degrees of relatedness. As policy ethnographer and medical anthropologist, my interest lies not with the complexities of the biochemical processes *per se*, nor do I take up here the thorny issue of (the mechanism of) 'internal agency' that has dogged molecular genetics from the outset. Rather, I draw upon the spatial idiom of translocation figuratively to question how it may serve as a point of chiasma between the natural and social sciences and inspire the rematerialisation of human biological form.[35] Specifically, I extend the term as a metaphorical and political field in order to explore the practices of knowledge operating both within genetics, and across the domains of science and ethics more generally. Following this cultural inflection, translocation allows one to explore the various interrelationships between error and chance, movement and flow, transfer and exchange that take place between regions and organisms, and also between places and people, where such regions are both figurative and material. What happens to the *chiasma* of biological translocation when it is conjoined with the anthropological tropes of displacement, relocation, diaspora and travel? To answer, it is necessary to give translocation a processual twist, and accordingly the metaphor can be transposed to consider its practical applicability in the context of various contemporary developments in the politics of genetics, especially the recent conceptions of so-called 'genethics' (see above, this chapter). Translocation, more specifically, becomes a matter of public accountability for scientists and non-scientists alike, and introduces questions that cannot be limited only to what persons inside remote laboratories take to be the usually invisible movements of alleles, chromosomes, proteins and genes.

Seen as an expansive linkage map and specialised 'tool' of its own, ethnography refers here specifically to the potential to mediate through translocation between the usually separate worlds of science and ethics. In the particular context of human genome technology and applications of genetic analysis discussed in this book, ethnography as linkage refers to the ongoing practices of translocation between the ethno-knowledges alternately represented as systems of 'fact' and systems of 'value'. But 'ethnography as linkage' is both a practical and theoretical movement that seeks to problematise rather than to achieve the promise of any smooth translation.[36] Stepping for a moment outside the conventions of the UNESCO meeting mentioned earlier, I take a small segment of what is potentially a wider ethno-ethical frame relating to genome research, so as to look again at certain connections between the two ethno-epistemologies: Western science and ethics. I am not suggesting that by good will and perseverance alone medical geneticists and cultural anthropologists can straightforwardly 'talk' to one another so as to render each other's assumptions transparent and 'translatable'. What I am suggesting is a narrower, more modest effort in which social anthropology is seen as a critical tool for assisting in degrees of critical conversational exchange that can modulate flexibly without loss of perspective between molecular and (ethno) ethical levels. The point, of course, is that within and between different disciplines, different levels of organisation and scale require different types of description and explanation whose metaphorical effects need to be made explicit in theoretical acts of

epistemological boundary crossing. Steven Rose (1997), as 'integrative' biologist of the neurosciences makes this point with his plural trajectory of holistic
'lifelines' and autopoietic organisms; and Marilyn Strathern (1991), from a different perspective as social anthropologist, has been concerned similarly with
the 'fractal' effects of domaining knowledge. A partial connection, Strathern
suggests, can dispense with questions of scale and proportion so long as the
analytic differentiation between comparison(s) is kept constant through the con-
tainment of detail. This is how, through the material and figural dimensions of
translocation, we can move sensibly between the expanse of continents and the
compressibility of chromosomes. Where we might see heredity as one local
model of genetic reproduction, in another instance it is the everlasting work of
circulation that brings to life a different local model of social reproduction.

Ethnography as a tool for linkage is also a directed intervention into the
temporality and ethics of doing field research in the context of a politics of
pre-emptive culture. We turn now to look at the emerging category of pre-
symptomatic rationality and the 'translocated' role of the anthropologist as
anticipatory diviner/ethnographer. Our conceptual interest will be guided again
by the question of why health professionals and those otherwise not customarily
engaged with anthropological reflection take heed of the ethnographer's insights
and the comparative linkage maps denoted by these revised 'translocations'.

PART II

'Home truths'

3

Foretelling foreknowledge

Verbal missiles and disclosure talk

People's accounts of dealing with the knowledge of inheriting HD can be described in terms of three key periods each involving the deliberation of multiple decisions. There is first the time of pre-testing deliberation and the decision whether or not to go ahead with the predictive testing protocol for those persons who have reason to believe they may be at risk of developing symptoms later. Second, the long-awaited day of the test result and the 'truth' of the revelation this brings. And third, the whole gamut of post-test experiences that mostly evade the follow-up work offered by clinically allied professionals. During the course of my fieldwork most people who had already taken the predictive test wanted to talk about the time they had first found out about their newly revealed pre-symptomatic status. Often, the rest of their accounts would fall into place around these narrated disclosures.[1]

Sam McDonald, a retired schoolteacher in her mid fifties, was one of the first testees who joined my research study. Reading aloud from her private diary, she recalls the day of her test result.

Well, this is what I wrote on the day of the result – you know, the day it happened. I was told today at the hospital that I had inherited the HD gene. I feel devastated and terrified. Dr P. was as always most concerned and supportive. Dr A. from the local clinic came to support me through the interview and see me home safely. I have been seeing Dr A. over the past eighteen months and he has been so understanding at all times. The degree of compassion particularly has been a lifeline to me.
Dr P. felt that there are many good reasons for not feeling too afraid. He said "If you were going to get it at any time in our history, now was probably the best time".[2]
Dr A. said that I should enjoy being well. I feel initially that I should redefine my understanding of hope. This has just been erased from my life and it is such an important ingredient. I do not regret my decision and playing dice with my life. I wanted the opportunity to be free of this disease [starts crying]. To gain thirty years

free from my anxiety and fear, emotionally I would have needed to be re-educated. I knew the devastating price I would have to pay if I lost. And I lost. So there we are.

Iris, a single woman in her late thirties, narrates in fast broken speech the moment the hospital-based genetic counsellor confirms what had been her worst fears.

I thought I was going to get a positive result. And I did. I thought I would be able to cope with it. [But] It's a living nightmare . . . it was a terrible shock . . . the day of the test result was very stressful . . . My partner Jason came with me to the hospital . . . we saw the consultant and the genetic counsellor . . . We were waiting and I could see the counsellor getting my notes with my name on it. It was all very close by. And then she says: "I'm not going to keep you waiting any longer. I'm very sorry, it's a positive result". Then we just sat there in the room. I think we discussed a few things. I can't remember exactly. She said something like: "How are you feeling?" And "if you want to come back, just call". And the hospital rang me, one week later.

The following is an extract from a personal account by Laurie, a university student, sent to me before our first interview meeting. It describes the day he and his brother, accompanied by their father and positively tested mother, return to the genetics clinic to learn their test results.

We arrived at the clinic at one o'clock. My brother and I were straight away taken into a room by the professor and his assistant. We all sat down and were told again of the general procedure making sure there were no misunderstandings. I was then taken to another room, identical to the first, two doors up the corridor. As soon as I sat down the professor told me my result and left the room to inform my brother of his result. I looked at the thick glass window, I looked at the door, I looked at the coffee table, I looked at the window again. The door opened. My brother came in. We walked towards each other and hugged.

I said 'So what's your number then?'
'18' he replied. 'What's yours?'
'41' I said . . . . '41'.³

We then joined our parents in the other room and spent 15 minutes behind closed doors to collect our thoughts and have a group hug. We left soon after and spent the next couple of days coming to terms with this new information. We knew it would be tough but at least now we know where we all stand.

It was the directness of many such accounts that first struck me when I began to listen to these divergent narratives of genetic revelation. Notable too was the fact these testimonies could not be heard as secular interpretations of intercession or religious symbolism. When people talk about the transformative potential of new genetic knowledge and contextualise such predictive knowledge directly in terms of their own lives, it is notable that they tended not to foreground religious factors within the moral compass of their decision-making.⁴ At first I was rather interested in the way that my research interlocutors seemed to speak with a somewhat resigned air, filling in here and there details about the day of the test result as something from the distant past, even when testing had taken place relatively recently. As the research study progressed and more families came forward enabling a broader picture to be built up, it became clear that participants were not simply passive recipients of information given to them by clinical professionals. Rather they were developing their own indigenous vocabulary of explanatory justification, integrity and vulnerability. Nor did these narratives necessarily conform to a view of biology as inevitable destiny, despite the autosomal dominant inheritance pattern of Huntington's as a single monogenic disorder. As we will see, many of the accounts were highly emotional, intimate kinds of kinship communication often ambivalently interlaced with sentiments of hope, contradiction and conflict that made them much more than simply the fateful testimonies of genetic futures 'already cast'. If on occasion it would also seem that families had experienced such clinical encounters passively as moments that had simply happened *to* them, then testees may have imagined other less obvious associations. Possibly it was through these narrations that they felt they could re-enact, and possibly cancel out, just momentarily, the detached professionalism that had characterised the clinical delivery of their irreversible result.

When Bronislaw Malinowki coined the phrase 'verbal missile' to denote the efficacy of magical words characterising Trobriand ritual speech he suggested that the conversion of 'breath' into strings of words with anticipatory effects enabled magicians to take speech out of the ordinary realm of everyday assertion. In this way hope and confidence could be generated for 'a morally integrated attitude towards the future' (Malinowski 1978:245, 248). The term *vatuvi* denoting a complex of magical acts is an example of a ritual word whose paradoxical and metonymical structure stands for an aspect of the whole situation yet whose referent cannot be translated in connection with any specific object or agency. Its linguistic and material power is pluripotent in the sense that it is 'rich in associations and reaching out in many directions' (248–9). For our purposes the comparison happens to be significant. As Malinowski describes it, the Trobriander would value the spell as a sequence of words whose magical potency has existed *ab initio* – from the beginning of all time. The spell of the magic – the sequenced string of words that are ritually performed – belongs to its own canon of socially transmitted knowledge, handed down between successive generations of specialist magicians even though beliefs about the origins of magic are inconsistent and unclear according to indigenous accounts (*ibid*: 214–17). As we saw briefly in Chapter 2, the substance of DNA, according to dominant scientific convention, is also discernible as a sequence of 'coded'

words made out of the basic units of the nucleotides: adenine, cystosine, guanine and thymine (A, C, G and T) and indeed molecular biologists happen
to believe that these are strung one after another in a long linear sequence
which makes DNA a molecule. We may see this scientific view likewise as yet
another local theory about the origins and reproduction of human life, albeit
one that simply happens to have stressed over everything else factors of biological transmission in its representation of objective 'fact'. What I simply want
to retrieve for the moment from this juxtaposition of alternatively arranged
'sequences', is my own ethnographic bearing in relation to acts of narrative. In
the biomedical encounter, it is sometimes the finality of the utterance – rather
than the words in themselves – as delivered by the mediatory figure of the clinical geneticist or counsellor that will transform a testee into a pre-symptomatic
person. This may well make this Westernised transposition to verbal missiles
a pretty unimaginative analogy, since the wished-for hope of a clear result –
the verbatim news that is delivered – metaphorically shoots through the person.
But the point is that the aesthetic is mediatory at all levels: information flows
or passes 'through' another site, person or entity. And in the critical disposition to assemble multiple stories from multiple sources, one could say
that the person of the bioethnographer – the anthropologist as the figure of
diviner – simply happened to be privy to the embodied effects of the figurative
'after-echo'.

Whereas for Westerners the process of scientific experimentation is founded
typically on the possibility of the recursive modification of objective knowledge over time, for Huntington's testees there is nothing cumulative about these
'one-off' highly subjective events of genetic revelation. Whilst the structure of
controlled experiments in sanitised environments allows the conventions of
science to refine, revise and even refute previous knowledge claims, possibilities for 'falsification' (Popper 1959) beyond the space of the laboratory are
not always a realisable strategy for reshaping the contours of the (genetic)
'truth'.[5] Thus the scientistic positing of data as provisional 'fact' within cultures of research experimentation contrasts with the 'finality' accorded to the
irreversibility of knowledge that is said to reveal somebody's genetic predisposition and future prognosis. The test result and the revelation it brings
for people is indeed a life-transforming event, but it is one that cannot simply be localised to the space of the clinic nor limited to the time of the
present.

Having received their results, many testees say they feel unsure what to say
and how to act with close kin and other social acquaintances. Making what
once seemed like ordinary and everyday decisions becomes a complicated and

demanding process of selection and evasion, even sometimes for those with supposedly 'good' news, that is, for those who have received a clear or negative result (see Chapter 5). But such pragmatic doubts underlie what is also a sub-narrative about the value informing pre-symptomatic classifications themselves. In her study of occupational therapy interventions in North American occupational therapy clinics, anthropologist Cheryl Mattingly (1998) argues that narratives are not simply retrospective accounts of past experience but are therapeutic 'emplotments' that guide and give shape to future action. To illustrate some of the processes of ethical deliberation in the contexts I describe, the following discussion considers how people emplot narratives of medical science and genetic testing as the anticipatory rituals of experimental technology.[6] We will consider how the 'genetic oracle' can be read and embodied as prophetic knowledge, explore whether its version of 'truth' always conforms to lived experience, and if not, how discrepancies may be contested otherwise as forms of moral knowledge.

Experimental technology as anticipatory ritual

People would usually offer many reasons why they had decided to go through the predictive testing procedure. There may be a sense that 'one's a bit different' or simply an intuition that 'there's something generally wrong', as Iris explains:

> One of the main reasons I had the test done was that I had a hunch I was positive . . . I was changing . . . not coping well with work, tired all the time, short-tempered, concentration was getting poorer, [I] was gradually backing off from friends. Everything seemed to be slipping backwards.

Parents or siblings would also talk about having hunches after one member of their family tested positive and opened 'a can of worms' that might implicate them. These 'best guesses' might only circulate as imagined probabilities insofar as certain kin (typically siblings) often will 'pre-elect' whom in the family they think might already be genetically predisposed, or what in kinship talk would be referred to as the next [person] to 'get it' (see Chapter 6).

For most clinical geneticists, obstetricians and genetic nurses overseeing DNA-based diagnoses, prophetic genetics is a 'science' far removed from intuitive hunches. Since the broad professional view holds that it is preferable in the case of so-called 'adult-onset' conditions for a person to know their risk

status than not to know it, an implicit prescriptivism underlies the entire regulatory complex of predictive testing despite the ideal of 'non-directive' genetic
counselling.[7] But as Lucy comments 'it is the fact that there is a test [that] is
the problem – it is because it exists that you have a choice to know what is
going to happen to you'. The consumerist model of choice may be a double-
edged sword here, even if the genetic counselling process rests upon a particular
logic that attempts to guide potential testees through the sinuous turns of pre-
negotiating an uncertain future. As Rayna Rapp (1999:62) observes, genetic
counsellors are seasoned bilinguals crossing fluently between all manner of
colloquialism and the more technical register of science-speak in their role as
information providers and risk communication 'brokers'.[8] Nonetheless the aim
of information provision does not obscure the fact that the counselling exercise itself rests upon some fundamental contradictions. As an information and
consent-obtaining process modelled on knowledge communication and acquisition, it turns on the expectation that a patient will be able to make rational
decisions whether or not to proceed with the testing protocol.[9] The genetic counselling profession presumes further that in order for 'client-centred' decision-
making to be seen as properly informed, people should be presented with all the
'facts' so that they can weigh up all the options and arrive at the 'best' course
of action. It is assumed, in other words, that potential testees themselves will
think they need counselling in order to be able to arrive at the requisite 'clarity'
of vision normatively prescribed by the regulatory complex. For many patients
and vulnerable persons, such support may be invaluable for helping them start
to explore the practical and emotional consequences of testing decisions that
confront them. Others may even request a more formal form of guidance and
'direction'. At the same time though some people may consider themselves
to be sufficiently informed about their family history or the nature of the condition for which they request pre-symptomatic testing. Is it then possible that
in certain situations some persons actively will prefer not to receive external
support through pre-and post-test counselling? Listen to Dylan, one of my
research participants, who commented angrily on what he took to be the inflexible requirements to undergo the protocol for genetic counselling prior to his
testing. He was indignant to learn the test would be denied him unless he agreed
to pre-test counselling.[10] His was just one voice amongst many critical of the
paternalism of the National Health Service:

> Health services don't always know best . . . why should I be subjected to this
> counselling? I'm in middle-senior management and I don't need someone telling
> me what issues I need to think about. And then you know, I mean it's just not right
> they left my wife out 'cos she stood to suffer the most . . . Why should they trawl
> through the baggage of my personal circumstances? Why?

Behind Dylan's protestations, we may ask related questions about the role and organisation of genetic health services. What kind of ethical system is it that fails to recognise that it is precisely because genetic testing candidates are 'human' that no counselee can be sure to know in advance the exact effects elicited by such foreknowledge for one's future well being and sense of self? This difficult question, presently evaded in the genetics counselling literature, looks set to become only more challenging for care providers. In line with the expected expansion of genetic counselling services particularly into the primary healthcare arena, it is likely that general practitioners (GPs) will assume a major responsibility for counselling patients in the coming years and for making referrals to other specialists. Recent recommendations for teaching genetics as an integrative discipline at all stages of professional education (see, for example, Department of Health 2003: 49–51) will need then to factor in the relevance of numerous socio-cultural differences across given contexts as part of an evolving training strategy for public health professionals. This is a pluralistic vision.[11] In the context of counselling, different professional contexts and different genetic conditions may evoke different degrees of need for 'direction' on the part of both clients/counselees and professionals/counsellors. Such variation not only speaks to multidisciplinary collaboration across and within different areas of expertise, it invites a fluid kind of professional reflexivity built upon the core value of flexibility. As Brunger and Lippman observe (1995:156) 'in the actual practice of genetic counselling, different individuals *do* need different information' which may involve the transmission of different 'facts' to different 'folks'. Managing people, managing relationships – it remains to be seen how such fundamentally anthropological endeavours will be negotiated by different teams of experts who are themselves governed by political ideologies of healthcare cost and measurement efficiencies.

Turning to those counselees who decide against testing, as well as those persons avoiding any direct encounter with genetic service care providers, I would often hear expressed the belief that 'only time will tell'. By deciding not to know more genetic information about themselves, this category of so-called 'at risk' persons effectively 'choose' an option that does not resolve their predicament since there can be no finality of knowledge that is gained one way or the other. They seek to avoid verbal missiles. Hermione's HD diagnosed father has been getting progressively weaker from the disease since her teen years and now in her late twenties she is definite she does not want to know whether she has inherited the same genetic disposition. Her relation to the present is shaped fundamentally by her prospecting of a future whose uncertainty creates what is only imaginable as the temporal deferral of prognosis. 'I don't picture myself reaching old age', she says. 'I try to make the most of my life now, being thankful for what I am able to do now. I don't want to put things off until the future because there may not be one'.

For others, pre-symptomatic testing is seen as a way of excluding oneself from the burden of a bad procreative conscience. It cancels what might have been manifest formerly as the parental worry of transmitting the disease to offspring. Several mothers and fathers with teenagers approaching the legal minimum age for testing would say it becomes important to 'spare' their children the trauma of 'direct' testing. This group of persons preferred to pre-empt the genetic status of their own biological heredity before offspring would be required to face similar decisions for themselves. As we will see, however, in practice the local kinship ethics of genetic decision-making construes the value of the pre-symptomatic person in radically different ways. The following extracts juxtapose accounts by Ruth and Dylan Jeffrys, a young married couple with two teenage children, and further reflections from Sam McDonald, a divorcee and single parent, to examine how decisions about predictive testing are 'emplotted' in future time as divergent moral relations between kin.

Ruth and Dylan Jeffrys

Recalling the events of one late summer's evening, Ruth describes how the family was enjoying a leisurely *al fresco* dinner in their back garden when Dylan received a telephone call from his father. Jake had rung unexpectedly to inform Dylan that his two grandchildren, Michael and Sandy, should know about a serious hereditary illness that may run in the family. Shirley, Dylan's mother, was not at all well and the doctor had come up with a diagnosis. Apparently it was something to do with her genes. Had Dylan ever heard of Huntington's?

The following extracts are from 'An uncertain future' – a diary journal and retrospective log of events written by Ruth. I intersperse here a few of the excerpts from Ruth's diary with some of the written comments and reflections of events offered by Dylan. Though Dylan chose not to keep a personal diary himself, he was moved to write down some detailed notes and comments once we had talked together about his experiences.

> After all the tests that his Mum had been undergoing, it appeared that she has Huntington's chorea. Armed with this information I had to look it up in our medical encyclopaedia – needless to say it wasn't listed under H but under C for chorea. Upon reading this information – that children have a 50–50 chance of inheriting the condition – it made for a very fraught evening. To say that one is devastated to find out that this condition is in one's family is an understatement.
>
> *(Ruth)*

A few days later there was a meeting at Dyl's dad with a doctor – ostensibly to discuss Mum and Huntington's in general. We didn't learn anything that our very basic medical encyclopaedia hadn't already informed us of. I was the only spouse at this meeting. I suspect that the rest of the family looked on my being there as an intrusion, but at this point in our lives we had been married for 17 years and given the nature of the Huntington's I felt that I very much had a right to be there – after all, if Dylan was to be one of the unlucky ones that inherits the Huntington's gene, he could pass that on to either one, or both of our children – and I then stood to lose all of my family. Not only lose them. But I would have to cope with watching them die over the years. I know it was not going to physically affect my own body but I would be the one that would have to pick up the pieces.

(Ruth)

In August 1996 my mother was diagnosed as having Huntington's. The diagnosis possibly now explains some of my mother's problems in the past. The diagnosis proved to be something of a solace to my father, who had to deal with the brunt of my mother's aggressive and violent behaviour, but to my two brothers and two sisters and I it was less than welcome news. We were told the main consequences of the diagnosis at a family meeting, in my father's house, convened to allow us to ask the geneticist any burning questions. I have to say that my immediate reaction was not to have to be genetically tested. You've asked me what emotions I felt. In the first two days after the news I felt a whole gamut of emotions – anger, frustration, vulnerability, self-pity, resentment, injustice, but these were just the initial response. I did some research into Huntington's and learned more about the disease . . .

(Dylan)

Dylan continues, introducing considerations about his son:

My wife and I discussed Huntington's at fairly regular intervals addressing the factors involved and the effects, or not, of genetic testing. There were far more issues than just a positive test, and whilst not being tested was my initial reaction it was obvious that there were more considerations than my own preference. As my son approached his 18th birthday and could therefore be tested, I decided that I would like to be tested and possibly save him unnecessary trauma.

And from Ruth's viewpoint:

We spent a lot of time talking about it. More to begin with obviously, then we just had to try to live with it. It was very hard and tensions ran very high at times.

Michael was coming up for eighteen, sexually active, so Dyl decided that he would take the plunge. The 'not knowing' was becoming untenable. It was a very hard decision for him to make. If it was positive he would be doomed to endure a living death – a very hard end for a bright and very physically active man, but on the other hand, if it was negative then his son would not have to be tested.

In her journal entries, Ruth goes on to describe the time between finding out about the presence of the illness on her husband's side of the family and the time when Dylan eventually went ahead with the test as 'a bit like living in limbo'.

> I always seemed to have to act as peacemaker. He was always on a very short fuse.
> The least little thing would lead to an upset of some kind. And of course, I would
> be thinking – is this a sign, something to do with behavioural problems? And every
> time he twitched in bed – is this it? And I know that the pressure he was under
> seemed to make him drop things – but was this it? I am a keen blood donor – and
> Dyl had done some to some extent, but he always seemed to have an excuse not to
> go – frightened that someone might find out something from his donation. He was
> also having problems with his shoulder – maybe this could be a sign?! So many
> little things that would normally pass unnoticed suddenly took on a new dimension.
> It is very hard trying to live under this strain. I would sit at work and suddenly a
> thought would hit you and you could feel the tears building up and you had to fight
> them down – how would one explain it?

Dylan, as it turned out, happened to test negative. However, as a descriptive vignette about the creation of a prognostic category of 'foreknowledge', the couple's own record of events shows up something of a grey area between the temporalised shadings of subjective 'illness' experiences. In nosological terms, there is an unaccountable liminal zone – or narrative 'gap' as Mattingly (1998:85) would say – between being 'a-symptomatic' and thinking oneself well, and being classified culturally as somebody who is potentially genetically verifiable as 'pre-symptomatic'. How one lives that uncertain zone as temporal experience, how pre-tested people negotiate the meaning of genetic foreknowledge for themselves and others, opens up a gap of time between fears of an anticipated diagnosis and the anticipatory constitution of the self as embodied prognosis. This gap of time, I am arguing, is a crucial cultural component of the making of the pre-symptomatic person.

Prognostic moralities

In *Death Foretold*, a book on contemporary American physician-internists specialising in 'internal medicine' (mainly oncology, cardiology and intensive care), medically trained sociologist Nicholas Christakis (1999: 197) describes prognosis as a 'sort of "future of the present illness"'. In so doing, the author begins an argument that denies a clear differentiation between the two knowledge systems of diagnostics and prognostics. Diagnostic evaluation – the ability to determine the nature of an illness and distinguish between illness classifications – is fundamentally prognostic in nature, he suggests, since the real cultural meaning of the finality of the diagnosis for both patient and practitioner lies in the articulation of clinical judgements about the future. To give a diagnosis is to create knowledge in the present about somebody's likely well being; and, from the patient's view, receiving a diagnosis is about having *already* some sense of one's movement forward into illness, even if this be a movement deeply resisted through pervasive denial. Now these assertions, if empirically sound, downplay the role of 'diagnostic supremacy' that characterised much of twentieth-century Westernised medicine. This is to say that when the ready availability of a cure dominated the medical repertoire, as the materialisation of the 'curative fix' through antibiotics and other life-saving pharmaceuticals, then matters of prognostication tend to seem as though they are relatively irrelevant concerns.

It is worth noting that a contemporary focus on prognosis is, in a sense, something of a renewed interest in medical prognostication that takes us right back, though not quite full circle, to the concerns of the Hippocratic practitioners of early Greek medicine. Not quite full circle because the link in ancient (5th century BC) diagnostics between prognosis and specialist medical knowledge rested quite singularly upon the healer's purported mastery of foresight regarding *acute* diseases. What we can see from an analysis of primary and secondary materials is how very human some of these ancient prognostic knowledge practices must then have seemed to physicians and patients alike. The emotions of fear and blame, feelings of personal worth, prestige and honour all come to the fore.[12]

In the genomic era, this collapsing together of diagnosis and prognosis is particularly evident once again in the shift towards the application of genetic testing technology, especially predictive tests. In explaining to prospective patients the differences between diagnostic and pre-symptomatic genetic testing, or carrier and susceptibility testing, clinicians and other health-related professionals are already inventing, enacting and legitimising the story of pre-dispositional monitoring as new political 'truths'. When inherited diseases are late-onset in their manifest symptomatology, the foreknowledge derived from such predictive tests makes genetic prognostication itself a fundamentally chronic affair. Uncertainty and subjective emotion prevail in expansive proportions, though for quite different reasons to the exculpation from self-blame sought by Hippocratic physicians, and indeed for reasons fundamentally other than those that trouble the physician prognosticators Christakis describes.

Identifying some of the powerful norms militating against the professional development and communication of prognoses in their general medical practice, Christakis (1999:185) suggests that physicians may be likened to 'reluctant prophets'. Prognostication is not just something that is avoided by doctors, but is a duty that is actively dreaded mainly because of the fear of doctor error through misdiagnosis or nondiagnosis, and also because of the portentous association between prognosis and death. 'To the extent that prognosis is linked with death, prognostication is necessarily mysterious, dangerous, and, there-fore, dreadful' (*ibid*, 186). This is not to withdraw Christakis' former asser-tion concerning the impact of a prognosis upon the meaning and finality of a given diagnosis, but rather to recognise that breaking bad news has never been easy for practitioners. In the age of genetic prognostication, it is now ordinary people who must live for many years with the anticipatory knowledge that they, as well as genetically related 'blood' kin, may be perceived as 'ill' (pre-symptomatic) before they are evidently 'diseased' (symptomatic). But what are the social and cultural effects of creating such foreknowledge amongst a new citizenry of 'moral prognosticators'? How do ordinary people manage prognostic fear as they disclose 'bad' news to others who may share with them a similar genetic inheritance? How do ordinary people make sense of such genetic foreknowledge?

That lazy summer's evening, Jake's telephone news changed everything. Simply on account of having to deliberate what action to take in relation to his disclosure of genetic information about Shirley (Jake's HD diagnosed wife), members of the Jeffrys family each assume – in different ways – what can be reckoned in cultural terms as a 'pre-symptomatic' status. The sheer decision of whether or not one takes action to know certain medical details about one's genetic heredity transforms an a-symptomatic person into the potentiality of a 'pre-symptomatic' person. The very worry of having to speculate whether a particular bodily twitch might be indicative of something more serious; just the anxiety of wondering whether or not to tell their children something about this before Dylan is tested – these are all 'symptoms' that make up the pre-emptive envisioning of anticipated illness, loss and dying. In other words, persons are no longer simply a-symptomatically 'ignorant' of certain genetic knowledge since relatives already have at hand the information somebody in the family may be 'at risk'. Of course, in these contexts it is the information itself that is the source of the contagion. For Ruth, news of Dylan's risky health status also transforms her, if only temporarily, into a risk-related affine. Before the test and up until the time of the test revelations she prognosticates herself as a changed social identity: what of her own future should she find herself related as an HD in-marrying wife and long-term carer? She may even end up as the mother of two genetically affected children, perhaps the sole family member and survivor not to succumb to the disease. What then?

Sam McDonald

Like the Jeffrys family, the fact that Sam McDonald is mother of a young teenage daughter proves significant in her weighing up of the decision whether or not to get herself tested. Sam and her husband divorced over ten years ago, and she has since lived alone as a single parent looking after Belinda, her only child, and holding down a demanding job. When she first realised the disease she, as a child, had witnessed her late father suffering from is one that is *hereditary* and therefore implicates her health status as well as her daughter's, she confessed to being 'absolutely devastated'. One day Sam invited me to her home for afternoon tea and a chat. In great detail she narrated how she had spent an agonising fourteen years living the future pre-emptively, and 'plotting out', as she said, her desired course of action. Only as Belinda was approaching her sixteenth birthday and prospectively coming of 'informational' age as a 'genetic' agent in her own right – as an 18-year-old able to request direct testing for herself – did Sam feel able to entertain the possibility of acting upon those long-thought out decisions.

MK: Can you talk me through what happens when you find out that your father's illness was HD and that this is a genetically inherited illness. What happens at this time?

SM: Well, I mean what was I thinking? The worst thing was this is all going to happen again. That it is going to happen to me after all that we have been through. That this is going to happen again, and my bloody daughter too. So the first thing I did was go and get sterilised and my sister did the same, so that was the first physical thing we did. Meanwhile I shook and stuttered, yes literally. I was constantly saying to myself, "How . . . how on earth are you going to deal with this? How?" With Belinda, I ended up making her too independent. "But what am I going to do about this? I am not going through all of this again. Not for anyone". I went to my GP and sat there, and he said "Sorry, I don't know what you are going to do Sam". And he photocopied everything he could find [on Huntington's], and he put it all through the letterbox and he said, "you know, if you think long enough you will find your own way". So I sat and sat and sat and sat and about nine months later I thought, "I don't have to live with this. I could commit suicide". And the moment I made that decision I was back on course and I got my life back in order.

So it wasn't just dealing with it, I had to make a positive decision about what I was going to do with myself in relation to this. And I even decided, I even collected huge syringes, and alcohol, and I filled up on razor blades and I filled up a whole drawer full of goodies. And they sat there and they are still in the loft now. And all I have to do . . . and that was it. And once I knew that I did not have to live with it then I could move forward, but I knew that it could happen. Therefore Belinda, she had to learn how to look after herself.

(Recording stops for a few minutes)

SM: You have also got to remember . . . you have also got to balance that against the time there was nothing doing with Huntington's. I mean that was the definite thing, that was as definite to me as having the test done and getting the bad result. Let me see what I wrote down about when I had the test done [flipping through a small lined exercise book on the table].

MK: Because you are living all that time from the seventies, through the eighties and into the nineties not knowing . . . .

SM: [interjects] Yes, and I deliberately did that . . . not knowing because I wanted . . . I thought if this comes out badly I might be forced into committing suicide and I have my daughter to bring up. Therefore if I didn't know and I could live with hope. It was having the hope. It was having the hope removed that was what I could not do with. And I thought once I get Belinda off my hands then it would be a different ball game. And it was. But there had to be some sort of hope in my head, because having not been there, then if I had had a really bad day as they do happen with all of this, because your mind locks into it, all those years of sorrow, then I might have ended up committing suicide, and I would never have forgiven myself for it. So I wanted to do things properly and I wanted them to be right. So this is when I got the result of the test. I wrote it on the day [picking up her diary notebook from the kitchen table].

MK: Sorry, if we could just go back a bit for a second. Because this is when Belinda is 16 now? Is that right?

SM: You see, the ball game had changed at this stage, and also, I then started thinking, well, now she's 16 . . . and I didn't have any childhood, so I want to retire at 50 and have an old age, but I didn't know whether I was going to have an old age. So at this stage I thought I need to go and find out whether I am going to have an old age, and as it turns out I am not. So that was the way I plotted all of this. So at the end of the 1980s I went to talk about Belinda and also to meet the people up at the genetic clinic, and rather liked the people I saw, and they were actually interested in my story. You must remember I never ever talked to anybody about any of this in all of those years. Except to close friends. And not [to] many of them because it wasn't something I could talk about easily or would talk about and you certainly didn't talk about it at work, you know, it was not on. But the worst person in all of this was me. The one thing I have protected all of my life has been my sanity which is why I work on the wisdom side, I think, because when you watch a man [referring to her late father] lose his sanity like that, it's the most precious thing in the world – most people don't even think about it – it is your sanity and I protected it as if it's pure gold. And I am going to lose it one day so I am going to protect it even more. . . . So I then saw Dr A. about all the testing and we had various consultations. He was smashing. Then I had to go over to the regional clinic where I met with Dr. P. about having the testing done. I said I just want to know if I am going to have any old age.

In Sam's case, the decision of whether or not to get herself tested entails detailed preparation work extending over the best part of two decades, the years during her thirties and forties. This extended process of actively facing her death and the lived uncertainties of not knowing whether or not she was pre-symptomatic was an agonising, tormenting experience. But it was also one from which she felt she could not escape. Prognostic uncertainty became an active part of everyday social engagement: it infected her relations with work colleagues and friends, and most immediately shaped her maternal identity and sense of parental responsibility towards her possibly 'at risk' daughter. Having witnessed during her childhood unforgettable domestic scenes of suffering connected with her late father's HD-related dementia, Sam, like Ruth and Dylan Jeffrys, realised that receiving a positive diagnosis is as good as verifying an unfavourable prognosis. In other words, Sam already had proficient foreknowledge about the meaning of foretelling, its implications for herself and her daughter. Unlike her genetic counsellors, though, she literally *embodies* the knowledge that a predictive test, as a diagnostic evaluation, is fundamentally prognostic. Moreover, she also knows that once a diagnosis is made explicit as open 'revealed' knowledge about her future health, such foreknowledge cannot be reversed: it can never be 'untold'. Without any available cure, a bad diagnosis/prognosis will never go away. Hence, her furtive strategising over the prior collection of 'goodies' in the loft: thinking foreknowledge means a 'way-out' was prepared well in advance should it ever be needed.

These temporal paradoxes are at the heart of what it means to live pre-symptomatically. Whilst the professional transmission of a delivered diagnosis collapses immediately into subjective prognostic meaning for the patient, there is on the other hand a huge temporal gap between diagnosis and prognosis that defines the making of the pre-symptomatic person. Into this gap are all the lived experiences between the revelations of diagnosis and the time of embodying one's prognosis as an obvious set of 'signs', or manifest symptoms. And yet it is the emergence of this temporal gap as lived experience that is so consistently overlooked by health professionals in the prophetic genetics field.

For Sam McDonald and Ruth and Dylan Jeffrys, moral decision-making and moral agency have less to do with absolutist questions of 'truth', autonomy and the objectivist revelations of the predictive genetic oracle, than with styles of contextual relating and specific social ties. Kin are far more concerned with dealing with knowledge in terms of what Lock and Kaufert (1998) describe as 'pragmatic' forms of body work, or as actions that can be directed towards what Taussig (1987), describing Putumayo healing practices, refers to as the negotiation of 'death spaces'. Crucially, Sam wanted to know whether she was going to have 'any old age' because this will affect how she goes about caring for her daughter and making other practical plans about her career, pension and retirement. Genetic prophecy as prognostic morality unfolds, then, as an emergent and relational ethics that is contingent on the centrality of 'redefining hope', and by extension one's relation to death and dying.[13] In the end Sam made a gamble and came out badly. As she puts it, she 'lost' all entitlement to the hope that has seen her through her years of uncertainty and thus becomes unconditionally 'pre-symptomatic': the test result medically reclassified her from an a-symptomatic person of questionable 'at risk' status to someone with irreversible prognostic foreknowledge. This same reclassification led in turn to Belinda finding out from her mother she too is no longer simply all that she seems: a care-free, apparently healthy a-symptomatic young woman about to go off to university. What, she asks, is she going to tell any future boyfriends?

Everyday genetics and the pragmatics of uncertainty

The above accounts illustrate how the 'ritualisation of optimism' (Christakis 1999:165–9) that characterises the fairly commonplace ellipsis of prognostication in the health professional's sphere of biomedical therapy has already become for some people part of an 'everyday genetics' that is lived outside of the moral space of the clinic. The preservation of 'hope' as something previously key to the medic's dilemma (or self-justification) of whether or not to make prognostic information explicit to patients, is now part of the moral responsibility redefining the meaning of 'relatedness' between persons who think they may share similar sets of genetically transmitted chromosomes. The professional norm to avoid prognostic specificity and leave a ray of hope, to communicate with patients through ambiguity and provisionality, to avoid committing what

Christakis (1999:109) condemns as 'prognostic abandonment', has filtered into domestic space, becoming part of the moral *habitus* and negotiated fabric of kin relatedness. Through the advent of predictive genetic testing technology, ordinary people too are being expected to step into the role of moral prognosticator. However, the role of prognosticator in such contexts is no longer simply a deeply moral one 'governed by obligations of truthfulness, disinterestedness, completeness, accuracy, and empathy' (Christakis 1999:185). The prognostic repertoire of human genetics, and the attempt to salvage strands of hope, looks more involute as a composite of ideals. This is because the communication of 'prophesised' futures is bound also to profoundly emotional 'roles' about how foreknowledge can be disclosed between and across the generations as parental or filial expressions of love. Once Michael and Sandy Jeffrys found out that their father had not inherited from (grandmother) Shirley an a-typical trinucleotide CAG expansion repeat – this having triggered Dylan's mother's predisposition to Huntington's – both siblings reproached their parents for not having told them sooner about Dylan's testing dilemma. Michael, the older sibling, especially felt resentful that his parents kept him in the dark about Jake's phone call on the evening his grandfather had rung. Belinda McDonald, by contrast, was profoundly annoyed with her mother for burdening her with genetic knowledge she did not want, and refused to say that this was information she would have asked for had she had the choice to know.[14]

Let me make at this juncture a link to an altogether different context. I want to introduce anthropologist Susan Reynolds Whyte's (1997) exposition of 'uncertain ethnography' on the health-related adversity experienced by the Nyole peoples of Eastern Uganda. This is a study dedicated in large part to what the author calls the 'pragmatics of misfortune' (Whyte 1997:224–6). Whyte describes some of the concrete everyday problems of social interaction amongst the Nyole, in particular the escalating incidence of AIDS and the evasive talk by locals about who has become a 'victim' of the illness. The pragmatics of misfortune, Whyte suggests, involves not only deliberating about things but acting upon adversity: those with illness are keen on 'trying out' (*ohugeraga*) a possible treatment or consulting a diviner to speculate upon or to test out who may have afflicted them and why. Such speculative behaviour is akin to a 'tactics of practice', Whyte argues (1997:216–17), since what people value is a form of consequentialist thinking that is one step removed from a broader philosophical framework on moral convictions about truth (see Chapter 4). 'Trying out is a hopeful, yet prudent, move that combines convenience with a realistic recognition of the uncertainties involved' (1997:105).

Like the Nyole who know misfortune by engaging with it directly, Huntington's families deploy social resources and personal experience to deal with various problems relating to their health and medical prognosis. Both populations appear to attempt to reduce uncertainty in terms of two key strategies: first, by mobilising kin in various ways (see Chapters 4–6), and second, by manipulating certain substances; in the case of the Nyole these are medicinal, rather than corporeal (see Whyte 1997: 229). My British interlocutors, however, also try to pre-empt the consequences of their actions as part of a more inclusive and deliberative process of moral decision-making. Further, these 'at risk' subjects find themselves governed by the cultural values of an emerging pre-emptive and socially discriminatory rationality. While the claim that 'knowledge resides in the consequences of directed action' (Whyte 1997:19 citing Dewey 1984:157) may hold well for the Nyole, the British families I describe can be said more accurately to 'test out' the experiences of *directed foreknowledge*.

Now it is precisely because these prognostic moralities engender such strong emotional registers that the lived 'gap' between anticipated diagnosis and embodied prognosis is time that cannot be narrated as a neat sequential chronology of remembered events. Pre-symptomatic temporality, in the fullness of its personal impact as lived meaning and cultural interaction, is not organised in narrative terms as a lineal progression of ongoing and anticipated suffering. As I try to follow Sam's train of memory and how she worked out the stages of her genetic decision-making as directed foreknowledge, I initially insert myself into her 'death space' through questions that attempt to situate intersubjective experience through a sequestered temporality. The nature of my interventions, however, reveals how my early orientation in this moral space has been guided partly by my own attempt, as empathetic witness, to map successively these illness events as a chronological sequence of sorts.

MK: Can you talk me through what happens when you find out that your father's illness was HD and that it's a genetically inherited illness. What happens at this time? (Intervention 1)

MK: Because you are living all that time from the seventies, through the eighties and into the nineties not knowing . . . (Intervention 2)

MK: So, if we could just go back a bit for a second. Because this is when Belinda is sixteen now? (Intervention 3)

Such questioning is a false superimposition by me, the researcher, of sequential time upon events and emotions that for Sam, and other participants, defied categorisation through lineal succession. How so? In the first phases of the conversation, I am trying to work forwards from the past to establish the accumulated sedimentation of foreknowledge, whilst for Sam the embodied knowledge of living life as a pre-symptomatic social identity is an all-engulfing constancy of doubt. The never-ending-ness that is the vulnerability of pain and the pain of vulnerability (cf. Kleinman 1988:56–74) charts a chronic space-time wherein the self is suspended experientially, caught in limbo between the expectation and outcome of what is already a foregone prognosis. There are no clear beginnings or endings to these layered stories of daily continuous uncertainty, though, as we shall see in the next example, non-sufferers cling to crude temporal measurements of 'before' and 'after' as a way of categorising the still 'foreign' classificatory entity of the 'pre-symptomatic'.

Lucy Williams

After several telephone conversations, the Williams family and I finally arranged the date of our first meeting. Prior to this, Lucy and I had spoken at length about the research and gradually she had divulged more about her personal link to Huntington's. She had taken the predictive test four years ago. That had turned out positive and Lucy said she now felt ready to meet me and speak at length face-to-face. She had heard about my research from a friend and wanted to contribute her views to the study. We were to meet outside of her home, she suggested, and her husband and two children, one of whom had also tested positive, had said they were keen to take part too. A few days before our meeting, I rang Lucy to confirm times and travel directions and mentioned that I had secured a room where we could talk in private without interference. Lucy sounded lively and said she was looking forward it. As this was to be my first at length interview with a family affected by HD, I was also hoping the day would go well.

Once we had said our hellos and settled down, Hanno, the younger son, suggested they each take turns to speak with me whilst the rest of the family would stroll around the vicinity. I was glad of his suggestion since I had been hoping to speak with everyone individually and then for all five of us to regroup towards the end of the day. Before the interviews proper were underway we went to a nearby cafe for coffee and I checked again whether, besides Hanno, everyone else was happy with a one-to-one interviewing arrangement. By the end of the day as we said our goodbyes, my overwhelming feeling of exhaustion – relating in no small part to the intensity of emotion that had accompanied these interviews – was alleviated only by a sense of surprise at how well our conversations had seemed to have gone.

The next day I left a telephone message for Lucy saying I would ring again soon. A couple of days later Lucy returned the call. She seemed annoyed. She was calling, she said, because she had been unhappy about having to wait in the cafe; it didn't have the kind of food she liked and had been too busy with excessively loud music. Besides, she went on, why hadn't I seen her limp, her walking stick and the other 'signs', and why hadn't I accommodated her needs more sensitively? I made my apologies as best I could but at the same time was taken aback at how narrow my field of vision probably must have seemed. Lucy had *looked* perfectly okay to me because she was an articulate and a vivacious narrator with a dry, sometimes hilarious sense of irony and playful humour. Somehow, these qualities had masked the fact that she already experienced slight *symptomatic* physical difficulties walking up and down a flight of stairs, making me at least temporarily oblivious to the full import of what it means to be somebody who is pre-symptomatic.

It was only when going back carefully over my tape-recording and the transcripts of our conversations that I was able to identify what I saw as moments of possible confusion and muddle in Lucy's account, though this in itself is hardly of particular noteworthy interest. What I realised more clearly was that much of what she had been saying related to her own attempted articulation of pre-symptomatic identity in terms of a local 'explanatory model' of genetic prognostication. This perhaps comes to the fore most clearly in a brief vignette describing her return journey home from the hospital on the day of the test result. Lucy and her husband, Rupert, had just dropped off to say hello to a close family friend and share with them news of the 'revelation' they had just received from the consultant clinical geneticist.

> The day of the test was quite funny . . .'cos, well, if you read my speech . . . Jack Paisley is a good friend of ours . . . Again you see we have this whole problem with friends . . . [cuts off]. Jack was in a state because they all came trundling out of the house, saying [imitating friend, exuberant emphasis]: "Oh, hi there! Well, do you have this, or you don't have this?", he's going, you know. He's very nice . . . very positive [imitating friend again]: "So you have this disease, or you don't?" I said, "Well, I do". "What do you mean you do?" [imitating Jack's disbelief bordering on exclamation], he says. "You do? Really?" [imitating incredulous surprise]. I said "Well, I probably don't, but, you know – I mean not yet" [hesitating tone]. "Look Lucy", he says [matter of fact tone] "do you have it or don't you have it . . . what is all this do, don't stuff . . .?" So you see I was confronted with this. And then his wife, Emilie is saying [imitating wife, anodyne, passive voice]: "You'll all be fine . . . You mustn't worry about these things . . ." And they're all talking at once. Everyone is talking at once. And I just went into a state of this is enough [gesturing with hands raised and outstretched before her]. I just wanted to go home, you know. Please. This is awful. So that's a kind of funny story now. I make it a funny story because it was. But umm . . . [breaking off] And then I suppose . . . after that, it's a kind of . . . after that your life *does* completely change and your whole family's life completely changes and it's this gradual, gradual change, you know. You think you're coping fine. And you're not. Nobody is coping. None of us are coping, you know.

Unlike the previous two cases, this third example captures a different sense of the prognostic momentum of 'foretelling'. Lucy's dilemma turns around the awkwardness of 'presenting oneself', in Goffman's (1963) normative sense of the 'public' self as person on display, as someone already knowledgeable of the fact she will become unwell in the future. Upon hearing of the test result, Lucy's friends find it difficult to place her legitimately within a pre-dispositional schema of pre-symptomatic personhood, just as I had done a few years on. Jack and Emilie responded to her attempt at illness revelation with incredulity, inadvertently dismissing Lucy's communication with the ritualised optimism of jolly rebuff: "You'll all be fine . . . You mustn't worry about these things . . .". The well-meant dismissal does not quite render the genetic revelation a non-legitimate fact, yet neither does it acknowledge the sense of pain nor vulnerability that is the undertone of Lucy's narrative. Then there is my oversight. Just beginning this particular field study, I was at that time still unfamiliar with the indeterminate language of anticipatory illness and the idioms through which people actively prognosticate their knowledge of heredity as future health. In effect, I had committed much the same *faux pas* as Jack and Emilie. Whilst conversing with Lucy, this researcher had thought no more of the odd linguistic slip up and had even welcomed her subject's narrative diversions as informative digressions. After all, as engaged fieldworkers, is it not towards such textured 'thick' digressions that most of us interested in narrative and life histories aim to work? As for Lucy's occasional pauses and my inaudible hesitations, I expect neither she nor I could have sounded more 'normal' an informant nor more 'inquisitive' a fieldworker. However, what differences there are that do persist between us cannot be effaced quite so easily from the written, worked-up and – according to the conventions – irredeemably 'objectivised' account.

Whilst I, as final authorial 'teller' of this encounter might choose to excuse myself (and thereby account for my own critical reflexivity in the field) by show-ing how theory making and confessing become impossibly intermingled, Lucy's narrative voice may be 'reclaimed' by seeing how she ends up [fore]telling a story within another story as a 'little therapeutic plot' (Mattingly 1998: 116–18).[15] Describing how the classificatory line between the categories of the pre-symptomatic and the symptomatic resists unambiguous differentiation as separate diagnostic entities, she inserted herself into the narrative frame by presenting herself as somebody suspended, almost imperceptibly, between the temporality of living pre-emptively (prior to testing) and living symptomatically (post-genetic diagnosis). 'It's this gradual gradual change, you know' she says as she reflects back upon the time that has lapsed between seeing her friends and the occasion that has prompted her now to talk with me. Narrative time has been organised within a 'gap' that assumes cultural meaning in terms of the awareness of how 'present events are configured by remembrances and anticipations – the concern to place the present within a remembered past and anticipated future' (Mattingly 1998:65). Lucy's disappointment that I had not been sufficiently perceptive of the subtlety of the corporeal shifts she was describing was as much a moral narrative about the cultural meanings attached to her prognosticated social identity, as it was a projected condemnation of me, the caricatured figure of the 'blind' researcher.[16]

Yet Lucy knew very well that her own 'explanatory model' of genetic prognostication was linked intimately to the corporeal foreknowledge she herself had come to embody. The concept of explanatory models (EMs) in medical anthropology, as originally devised by Arthur Kleinman (1978), has generated theoretical debates around the etic constructs of disease, illness and sickness, and their relation to 'nature' and 'culture' respectively (see critiques by Frankenberg and Leeson 1976; Taussig 1980; Young 1982; Hahn 1995). Kleinman suggested an EM is a set of beliefs encompassing any or all of the five features: aetiology, onset of symptoms, pathophysiology, course of sickness (severity and type of sick role) and treatment (Kleinman 1978:87–8). By identifying healthcare systems in terms of the different EMs deployed by practitioners, patients and family members, the medical anthropologist could establish a theoretical basis for cross-cultural comparison since, as Kleinman maintained, these EMs are located in all societies. Rather than repeat these well-rehearsed debates, I would suggest that at least so far as the new genetics is concerned, the concept of 'explanatory models' may be usefully revised by transposing, in the first instance, a little from Whyte's Ugandan materials on health and misfortune. Whyte suggests that the Nyole cannot always distinguish between sources of uncertainty and the means of dealing with uncertain events (Whyte 1997: 204–5): what the author calls 'extrospection' and 'relational power' refers to the agent's plural identities and relationships dependent on context. I would suggest likewise that clear distinctions between the categories of pre-symptomatic and symptomatic illness, and the related classifications of 'diagnostic' versus 'predictive', is more an illusory than an accepted way of knowing for most of the research participants I interviewed. More profoundly still, there is the epistemological consideration that the creation of new categories of pre-symptomatic persons, again specifically in these particular 'high technology' contexts, radically challenges the Western biomedical notion of the patient as someone necessarily isomorphic with a presenting illness or cluster of detectable symptoms.

Lucy knew she embodied the seeming cultural paradox that is inherent in living life as a 'pre-symptomatically symptomatic' person. Feeling her symptoms to be real, yet aware that to others these appear not 'real enough' to be visible as outward signs – and herself not really sure of when precisely she had slipped from one state of symptomatology to another one more manifest and clinically serious – Lucy's illness experience is replete with prognostic uncertainty. It is this sense of an inconclusive and elusive sickness trajectory that makes the narrativisation of her therapeutic plot fundamentally 'little'. As a 'halting, skeptical, little narrative' (Mattingly 1998:116), Lucy's account overturns the formal structure of the grand narrative replacing the sequential progression of events with an emplotted 'foretelling of the self'. Shunning any sense of the illness episode as one marked by clear identifiable beginnings and endings, diagnosis and prognosis have fallen into each other.

What does it mean to be 'pre-symptomatic'?

In each of the three cited examples, we see that a protracted and agonising period of 'knowing about not knowing' gives way to the decision to have oneself tested and thus to have revealed the 'truth' of one's biological make-up as the irreversible knowledge of a genetic inheritance. Paying close attention to the lived value of social identity as temporalities of embodied prognosis, the commentary has suggested that it is necessary to question the analytic demarcations set up by the classificatory markers of the 'pre-symptomatic' versus 'symptomatic'. I have pointed to how key evaluative criteria, the 'diagnostic' and 'predictive' tools through which medical science attempts to classify people, are at odds with the way individuals and families over time provisionally 'test out', and painfully make sense of, the emotional work invested in local moralities of disclosure-as-prognosis. For an ethno-ethical knowledge link we can transpose a little from Whyte's Ugandan materials on health and misfortune and the suggestion that the Nyole cannot always distinguish between sources of uncertainty and the means of dealing with uncertain events (Whyte 1997:204–5). I suggest likewise that clear distinctions between the categories of the pre-symptomatic and symptomatic illness and the related classifications of 'diagnostic' versus 'predictive', is more an illusory than a pragmatic way of knowing for a number of the British informants with whom I conversed in my/our capacity as co-interlocutors. The inability of friends and others to grasp what 'pre-symptomatic' carrier status means, the failure to acknowledge an invisible but 'present' illness, like my own oversight with Lucy, or Ruth's 'watching' of Dylan, casts doubt on the biomedical distinctions between categories of the pre-symptomatic and their homological correspondence with the positivistic tools of prediction and diagnosis. The ethnographic evidence illustrates therefore that the subtleties pertaining to the category of the 'pre-emptive' as the lived experiences of predispositional persons are liable to be under-recognised and given sleight of hand culturally. As mentioned, these classificatory difficulties, and the epistemological problems they raise for illness categories and the social management of health generally, were brought directly home to me when, at the outset of the research, I happened to overlook how one research participant was already in the early stages of illness. My oversight evokes again the difficult problem of the 'invisibility' of chronic pain from the patient's perspective, and the associated 'de-legitimisation' of subjective pain experiences as a-typical or undiagnosable illness events that keep evading successful knowledge construction (Good *et al.* 1992, especially Kleinman's chapter pp. 169–97; see also Frankenberg 1992). Additionally, though, my oversight with Lucy Williams prompts recognition of another problem of knowledge perception. In thinking through what it means in cultural terms to create pre-symptomatic persons as a new classificatory order of (fore)knowledge, the fundamental question is *how* we think about whether or not we actually want this kind of prognostic information in the first place. And here's the rub. There is no such thing as prognostic information *per se*, only different categories of information that generate different prognostic fields for the momentum of potential knowledge disclosure (Konrad 2003c).

The question of what information is transmitted in and through the medium of an 'anticipated prognosis' can no longer be limited to the exclusive domain of the physician, understood as the professional's acts of 'inward' and 'outward' prognostication, of foreseeing and foretelling respectively (Christakis 1999:192–4). Instead, such anticipations extend to, and indeed shape the very realm of 'true prognosis', or what Christakis simply defines but omits to study as the patient's own lived experiences. By understanding better how family members themselves share and communicate genetic foreknowledge as impending 'revelations' of death, as opposed to the reluctant divulgence of information by physicians or genetic counsellors *to* patients, we see how pre-symptomatic persons deal with the interval between the time of diagnosis and the materialisation of illness. We are able to start to understand how this constitutes an ongoing process of *embodied prognosis*, and therefore what it means to inhabit the worlds of the pre-symptomatic. By way of conclusion, I summarise the relevance of such expanded knowledge fields for the classification of different categories of prognostic information.

(1) Moral prognostication as an expansional field of knowledge generation

If a shift from the prognostication of clinical judgement to the 'prophetic' revelations of genetic tests alleviates certain burdens of responsibility for clinicians as 'reluctant prophets', then this also opens up a new arena for moral negotiation within and between family members. Ordinary people as kin relations become moral prognosticators, caught up in complex decision-making over the meaning of genetic information for their own and others' health futures. With the advent of multi-factorial genetic testing, such health communication will be extended in the future to moral choices in lifestyle and the modification of habits as the responsibility of the 'at risk' person.

(2) Foreknowledge itself as a model of chronicity

As people anticipate their futures in terms of certain 'what if' disclosure dilemmas, moral prognostication entails a continuous rehearsal of perceived risk susceptibilities. Foreknowledge itself is coterminous with, and embodied as, a *non-biological* modelling of chronicity.

(3) Patients have different tolerance thresholds for prognostic information

Not everyone will always want to access all the information that is potentially available about their genetic constitution: 'patients' and those a-symptomatic persons who are currently undiagnosed will have different desires and needs for prognostic information. This is a crucial point that underscores the importance of acknowledging that different family formations (and family members) will have divergent versions of what is to be gained from prognosis, especially in situations without effective therapy where no known cure or drug regimen is available.

(4) Looking poison in the eye: information as a source of contagion

Unwanted information, linked to point (3) above, may effect a prognosis in the form of a self-fulfilling prophecy. The disclosure of certain information may 'save' lives (or prevent some babies from ever being born), but equally, what for some persons is embodied as *too much* information, can do untold harm (see Christakis [1999:109] on the perils of 'terminal candour' and associated 'truth dumping'). The expedient use by doctors of prognostic uncertainty as a basis for optimism (managing prognostic information through provisionality and by leaving 'a ray of hope') passes now to the role of kin in the form of learning to know and embody the value of ambiguous speech. In certain situations it may be that those with the strongest kin connections feel impelled 'to care not to know' (and thus not to generate new diagnostic information for others) through intuiting the meaning of saying nothing. This could be an important consideration for health communication campaigns and public health genetics education training programmes in the future.

(5) Genetic agency as relational foreknowledge

It follows that the act of turning foreknowledge into explicit 'knowledge' as socially transmitted information is fundamentally a relational act. Information stands in relation to people in their capacities as relational agents. Thus, one person's genetic foreknowledge may be another person's non-knowledge in terms of what has not been disclosed.

(6) The limitations of *gnosis* as epistemological framework

The difference between diagnosis and prognosis cannot be served universally by the central epistemological template of *gnosis*, rendered in the Western medical repertoire as expertly defined knowledge systems of objective 'truth'. There can be little convincing conceptual need to rehearse the rightly much-critiqued rationalism of the post-Cartesian body[17] as (just) one version of disembodied 'ethno-knowledge', except to say that our own Western etymological roots in ancient Greek medicine are epistemological roots we have never successfully completely shaken off. Naturally this has far-reaching consequences. *Gnosis*, the Greek word for the act of knowing, happens to be conferred in practically every biomedical encounter through the dual conventions of first giving 'the *dia*gnosis' and then foretelling 'the *pro*gnosis' (as the knowledge that comes before ['pro'] the expected illness outcome). As we will see in the next chapter, understanding why people may prefer not to care to know genetic inheritance futures may yield forms of knowledge that are in some sense prior to other more 'scientific' forms of understanding. A renewed bioethical analysis in terms of the interrelations between 'interest and emotion' (cf. Medick and Sabean 1984) for concepts of genetic relatedness may shed further light on these issues.

4

Tracing genealogies of non-disclosure

Dilemmas of truth telling in conventional bioethics

Despite the declared ideals of 'non-directive' genetic counselling, testees with a detected predisposition may often find themselves encouraged by practitioners to believe it would be best to inform direct 'blood' relatives they too may face a shared risk of developing future illness. This purported 'obligation' to disclose genetic information to other family members is, however, more presumed an ethical virtue than an indigenously formulated kinship duty people themselves are moved to articulate (see Suter 1993; Zimmerli 1990; Higgs 1998; Jackson 2001).[1] Moreover it is one underscored institutionally by converging debates in mainstream biomedical ethics on the social responsibility or otherwise of the clinician to commit so-called 'unsolicited disclosure'. This latter principle evolves out of a particular rationale of decision-making that seeks to identify those circumstances in which it may be presumed right to disclose information that is genetically relevant to a relative (for example, siblings and cousins) without the prior consent from the original testee.[2] In this sense, unsolicited disclosure to a third party sets up moral dilemmas that quite obviously divide persons. On the one hand there is the assumption of the testee's right to privacy, and on the other the competing interests and assumed right of untested kin, as prospective recipients of genetic information, not to be told. The absolutist view that there are no instances justifying breaches of medical confidentiality appears to be mitigated by the more widely supported stance, endorsed in the UK by the General Medical Council, that exceptions may be permissible in cases where somebody else will be protected from serious harm.[3]

Such concerns have been subsumed most usually by the set of issues discursively framed in the bioethics literature as the 'right to know' and the 'right not to know' debates. Bioethicist Ruth Chadwick's (1997) important overview has identified three different possible claims for asserting the existence of rights with

regard to genetic information. First, the right to know one's genetic constitution and the relevance of such information for reproductive choice. Second, the
right of a 'third-party' to know the genetic constitution of another (for instance
claims made by partners, spouses, or by children in relation to parents). Third,
the right of institutions to know genetic information about individuals (where
claims to knowledge access may be based on commercial incentive or justified
by social ends, such as communitarian interests). Arguments for a right not to
know may span self-determination claims, or turn on consequentialist forms of
reasoning that posit likely benefits against harms, or seek to uphold the concept
of inviolable privacy. Summing up the positions, Chadwick's argument is that
there can be no simple opposition between a right to know/not to know on the
one hand, and between a right to know and a duty to know on the other. She
correctly suggests that conflicts of interest between different persons' right to
know and not to know may turn upon different types of genetic information and
conditions.

Taking a strong culturalist line, I want to suggest that this philosophically
determined dilemma about rights to knowledge/non-knowledge is noteworthy
not simply for its particular reasoning – namely, the consequentialist driven logic
that attends to the balancing of benefit against harm, the principle of beneficence
against the principle of maleficence. I want to show why the dilemma is noteworthy too for the particular social relations it elicits and 'stands for'. Whilst
these 'right to know/right not to know' debates raise several far-reaching ethical, legal and philosophical issues (Chadwick et al. 1997; Marteau and Richards
1996), it is important to see that the dominant conceptual framework for these
discussions is one modelled on the primacy of individual rights.[4] The pre-
cept of autonomy and associated ideals of confidentiality, privacy and freedom
underpinning this individualist premise however are at odds with the increasing recognition by professionals and policy advisors that genetic information
can never simply be information of relevance to one individual person' only.[5]
The British Medical Association has acknowledged the 'interrelatedness of
interests' between kin noting how '. . . although society puts great emphasis
on individual rights, the concept of a purely personal decision meets a great
challenge in the sphere of genetic knowledge and genetic technology' (British
Medical Association 1998:24, 26). Similarly a report on genetic screening by
the Nuffield Council on Bioethics (1993:4) notes that 'genetics and diseases of
genetic origin inescapably involve families' and raise 'some of the most serious
issues' in terms of the disclosure of genetic data between kin (1993:42; cf. Advisory Committee on Genetic Testing 1998). A prominent 'gap' in the bioethical
literature is opening up therefore between acknowledgement of the ramifying
effects of genetic information for consanguineal (and non-consanguineal) kin

on the one side, and the analytical and conceptual frameworks that underpin the development of a responsive bioethics and genethics discourse on the other. Moreover, the contours of this gap appear to be magnified yet further by the discrepancy between stories that come to the clinic and those that get told in the field. Since the 'right to know' debates that inform mainstream bioethics literature and policy in this area have not been built up in the first place from people's own experiences, it is important to see how divergent kin with different knowledge interests define and negotiate their own constructions of moral 'value'.

Since many anthropological materials have considered how indigenous forms of ethics and disclosure take place within a context that is far wider than the patient's right to medical information and the healer's obligation to provide it, the first point concerns the considerable medicocentrism of a tactics of truth disclosure. The second, 'truth telling', as a clinically based biomedical event, is embedded in particular relations of authoritative power and restricted access to knowledge whose 'therapeutic plot' (see Chapter 3) conventionally unfolds as the unilineal passage of 'truth' from the doctor or counsellor (presumed expert) to the lay patient (presumed non-expert).[6] What happens then when knowledge flows in other directions through the entangled webs of family secrets? As so little detail is known about how kin make moral decisions concerning genetic health outside the confines of the clinical setting, this chapter discusses the effects of predictive testing technology in terms of certain moralities of truth-telling and disclosure tactics. This analytic framework allows us to consider how telling 'the truth' is narrativised as reflexive processes of 'negotiated relevance' between kin, and further how these moralities may be diffracted through a wider 'ethno-ethics' of embodiment and knowledge.[7] To this end, we will trace some fragments of a genealogy of untruths as certain 'complicities of non-disclosure'. We will ask also a related question: 'What does the artefact and method of "genealogy" look like when framed in terms of the non-knowledge of certain secrets embodied and transmitted over time?' Now the relevance of this approach might not be immediately apparent to non-anthropologists, but in fact it is directly germane to the practice of genogram construction deployed by numerous genetic counsellors and others. In session, genetic counsellors typically proceed to (re) construct genetic information as though fragments of personal life history may be amassed as totalising knowledge for the 'interpretive' truth designs that are 'elicited as' critical discursive tool: namely, the patient's own narrated medical pedigree. For their part, social anthropologists have always had a special affinity with genealogy and genealogical knowledge construction. At the beginning of the twentieth century genealogical information had been apprehensible to anthropologists as 'bodies of dry fact' (Rivers

1914; cited in Bouquet 1993:37). Rivers 'genealogical method' (1910) rendered the social recognition of biological ties a scientific class of abstract genealogical information and the family tree, as Mary Bouquet (1996) argues, became part of a visual language that made the illustrative genealogy an obvious artefact of kinship. This visual language was mined by science at just a time when ethnology's institutional insecurity happened also to make the pseudo-scientific guise of kinship look something more serious, more respectable and worthwhile. Of course the legitimisation today of anthropology within the academic and wider world is not usually thought to depend primarily upon the insights of contemporary kinship study. But what one might now see as renewed theoretical interest in kinship – occasioned in part by recent critiques of the new life technologies – could be said to be one of the reasons why scientists and medics might seek to 'extract' new genealogical data from the vantage of contemporary social anthropology.

Embodiment and moral knowledge

The Opie family

By the time I first met Daisy Opie in 1998 she had taken the test for HD and had tested positive. In her mid-20s, she was mother to three young children, Jamie (aged five and half), Rosa (aged three and half) and Penny (9 months). Gregg Duggan, the children's biological father, had been cohabiting with Daisy prior to the birth of Jamie, and each partner independently furnished me different reasons why they had not 'tied the knot', Greg particularly summoning up reasons why marriage had been deferred. For her part, Daisy proclaimed to know much of what to expect for her future, having herself witnessed her mother's chronic degenerative illness over several years. Much of this foreknowledge was narrated in terms of how secrets had formerly circulated as particular kinship relations within her birth family.

It had been under the convenient euphemism of 'Mary's nerves' that Jack, Daisy's late father, had managed to withhold from her and her elder sister, Liz, the diagnosis that the medics had disclosed to him many years earlier, sometime in the 1970s about his wife, the siblings' mother. During their teenage years, Jack had also kept up other false appearances covering over 'for the sake of his children' the extent of the difficulties he was facing as Mary's sole full-time carer. Daisy subsequently learnt that the formal diagnosis had taken place many years earlier than she had first been told and to this day remains aggrieved her father complied with the doctors by withholding from her the 'true' extent of her mother's illness. Yet this is a 'grievance' that is not recounted by her as a breach of a relation, but as the forging of relatedness between Jack and herself. Each relative has used knowledge of the familial illness in similar ways – to keep from the other what each perceives father and daughter would extract from the situation as undesirable knowledge. Once Daisy is informed of her 'predictive' result, she is unable to tell Jack she has tested positive because this would have been 'devastating news' that would have put, she conjectures, 'the final nail in the coffin' for him. Father and daughter both were to worry about the other's future health, each implicitly recognising that the effects of the disease cannot simply be attributed aetiologically to genetic heredity and physiological likeness alone.

DO: I think he felt as if he wanted to talk to me more than was good. He didn't want to pull me into this carer thing, he didn't want that for me. I think that's what he was telling me, that's what it was. He didn't want to ruin my life by telling me, you know. I never told him that I'd had the test. I mentioned that the test was available . . . umm to see what his reaction was. He didn't want me to have it, and if I did, he would rather not know.

MK: So he never knew?

DO: As far as I know, I don't think he knew, no. I thought he'd suffered enough going through it with Mum. I thought it would be the end of him, for me . . . [breaks off]

MK: And you decided to keep this knowledge to yourself?

DO: I think he would have been very distressed. I think it would have been like . . . the final nail in the coffin, you know. I don't think he would have coped with that at all. I think it would have been devastating for him. It was devastating enough losing the wife that he obviously loved to bits.

MK: Would you say that you were looking after your father by stopping this knowledge? By not letting it go any further. By not telling him?

DO: Probably the same way that he protected me, you know (chuckling, nervous laughter). I think he was wrong in doing that, but like, because of the way, you know, he did it. Because he thought he was protecting me, which came out of one hundred per cent love. But I don't think it was the right choice in the long run.

MK: Has it made you think about the whole issue of how knowledge is used and . . .

DO: [cuts in] That's why I had the test done.

Is Jack committing a lie and deceiving his children by not telling them what he knows to be the case about Mary's health? Is Daisy committing the *same kind* of lie and deceiving her father by not disclosing to him the results of her positive test? To what extent does each party 'owe' the other the truth? And what about Mary's own views on the value of truth telling? Though Daisy's mother is conspicuously absent from the narrative, she nonetheless summons a vital presence since it is around her very person that these kin relations, as embodied ethical dilemmas, come to be created and recreated over time. Daisy says she acts to shield her father 'in the same way that he withheld information from me about mother'. Yet for each of them kinship emotion assumes a different kind of moral 'value'. Through her own act of concealment it is impossible for Daisy to 'return' the same kind of (non) knowledge to Jack because the value of 'unsolicited disclosure' is always context-dependent: it is always a matter of specific relations. Jack is positioned as the in-marrying spouse and primary breadwinner whose relations with Mary grew out of their shared affinal non-knowledge of her health status as 'pre-symptomatic'. Daisy, however, *knows* she is a positive HD carrier and that her future turns partly on the way she will embody herself as a female source of maternal procreative power (see Chapter 6). In other words, knowledge between kin travels with different moral valence: in this example persons in the form of an in-marrying father and pre-symptomatic daughter are divided into newly engendered relations of illness susceptibility.

But it is also clear that Daisy is not invoking the rational bioethical register of 'balancing' benefits and harms. Her calculations of 'best interests' originate from what we can see are the sheer inconveniences for her of truth telling. It is rather considerations of care and kindness to Jack – not wanting to hammer 'the final nail in the coffin' – that seem more relevant to her than the disassociated norm of straight talk imbibed in the principle of honesty. The activation here of 'untruth' as concealed non-knowledge recalls philosopher Sissela Bok's (1982:6) comments on the shared etymological origins between discretion and secrets. *Discernere* and *secernere* both refer to the activity of separation, to the ability to make distinctions. If the capacity to discern refers to the ethical activity of separating out things, the secret is that which *has been* set apart: it is hiddenness both as the form and the morality of 'set-apartness'. When Bok speaks of the 'active attention' that is required to keep things secret and of the 'countless shadings of belief, vacillation and guess-work' between knowledge and non-knowledge (Bok 1982:10), we in turn can say that Daisy and Jack 'discern' honesty as different kinds of perpetrated kin-ship secrets. In other words, both go about setting apart the truth in divergent ways. Where Bok's equation of secrecy as 'intentional concealment' (1982:5–7) falters, however, is in its presumption of fully charged-up volitional agents capable of recognising the various permutations that these 'countless shad-ings' of vacillation somehow assume. For both parties, concealment of certain knowledge has occasioned certain untruths but neither person has really *meant* to lie.

The Opie family's predicament raises the issue of how family secrets – as an ethics of kinship disclosure relating to human genetics – may involve different *degrees* of deception, discernment and truth reckoning. Some philosophers and ethics commentators, partly taking their cue from the positivist critique of Nietzsche (1873) have suggested that deception is endemic to daily life and furthermore that truth itself is an illusory ethical attainment (see Nyberg 1993).[8] F. G. Bailey's (1991) anthropological discussion of the ubiquitous prevalence of deceit in almost all realms of politics offers a qualifying variation of this post-Enlightenment theme with the claim that 'collusive lying' is homologous with the generation of 'open secrets' (Bailey 1991:33–4; 35–64). The view that 'collusive lying involves at least two parties who know what they say or do is untrue but who nonetheless collude in ignoring the falsity' (Bailey 1991:35) may be seen as a critical counter to Bok's (1979) earlier work on the ethics of secrecy and 'clear-cut lies'. Bailey's own ethnographic example from the Kond Hills in western central Orissa (North India) concerns the public pretences informing local marriage ceremonies and bridewealth speeches from the late 1950s. He suggests that the highly stylised and formal tone of these speeches conceals the prior behind-the-scenes talk during which time representatives from the two families will have agreed *already* what is to comprise the bridewealth and dowry exchange settlement. It is principally because of the enacted 'pretence' that the families are strangers meeting for the first time (the 'open secret') that Bailey concludes these ritual ceremonies can be perceived to constitute a falsification of a kind (*ibid*:38–39). Of course much greater critical elaboration of Bailey's own position as situated ethnographer would be required to develop the merits of this particular line of kinship disclosure as narrated experience. As it happens, the reader is offered just a couple of exemplary one-liners from the speeches for the defloration of the bride. Nonetheless, what is revealing in ethnographic terms about the Orissa example is how the drawn-out processes of negotiation informing decision-making, bargaining, compromise, confusion and disagreement between divergent kin have been *written out* of the local marriage record. The story of how these kin once were fictive 'strangers' does not become part of the conventional body of ritual folk knowledge and is denied temporal transmission across the generations as official history.

Jack and the consultant neurologists have also kept between themselves a kind of 'open secret' about Mary's diagnosis. In this case, the pretence that nothing had been detected medically can be sustained in part by the corporeal fiction of the 'deceiving' body that conceals its hereditary illness as pre-symptomatic time. Hiddenness is located in the corporeal person whose 'set-apartness' cannot be readily discerned. Rather than talking in terms of ubiquitous deceit then, which after all sets up what is simply yet another antagonistic and unhelpful dichotomy of 'truth' versus 'un-truth', we are in a position to reflect further how an ethics of kinship disclosure lends itself conceptually to a 'family' of untruths. The following sections continue to consider such kinship reckoning by exploring the sense in which different degrees or intensities of untruth also comprise contested versions of what can count as genetic veracity.

The Daley family

According to Isobel, getting married was something that 'just happened'. She and her husband Bruno Daley had first set eyes on each other in their late twenties after a 'one-off' chance meeting. A joke between Isobel and one of her friends had led to a blind date set up through a matching agency in town in the late 1980s. The couple got on well together, became engaged and it was not long before their first child, Stefan, was born. Then, over the next few years, Bruno, a senior business executive for a public relations company, started to slip up at work. Just small things at first like arriving late or missing appointments. He was probably tired and under stress, Isobel thought. Meanwhile the couple conceived their second child, Louisa. She was born roughly around the time when Bruno had started to receive a string of written cautions from his employer. This was followed by a demotion . . . the slip-ups had become professionally inexcusable.

Today, just approaching his fortieth birthday, Bruno spends most of his days confined to a wheelchair. With speech reduced mainly to monosyllables, it is now only football on television that can hold his attention for more than a few minutes at a time. As Isobel fills in the details of her husband's progressive physical deterioration, her account unfolds as the story of the transmission of genetic secrets between estranged kin. What had happened was that Bruno's estranged father Oliver had come across a long-forgotten death certificate containing post-mortem details of the likely cause of death of Bruno's paternal grandfather. The search for this document had been initiated by Oliver who had been feeling unwell and was worried about his increasing irritability and forgetfulness. On the advice of his general practitioner, Oliver had taken various steps to discover the details of his family's medical history. The doctor subsequently advised he should get back in touch with his ex-wife, Susie and inform her of the situation. Susie then called a family meeting at which she informed her children they best seek medical advice about the possibility they may have inherited an illness from their father. But Oliver's written 'disclosure' arrived too late for Bruno and Isobel to act on this knowledge. Once news of

Oliver's condition had reached them Isobel was already pregnant with their second child and decided against prenatal testing. Casting her mind back to the 'family meeting' her in-laws orchestrated in early 1992, she describes the moment they broke the shattering news of Oliver's letter.

ID: Well, we were staying with my in-laws and when I look back his mother was faffing around and she obviously was upset about something. We were thinking about making tracks to go back [home]. Anyway she kept saying "Stay for a coffee, please do" and so we did until Pete, Bruno's stepfather, came home. And then he came home . . . and he said, "Well, you do really need to read this". He was holding up a letter in his hand. Waiving it about. It was from Dad. "Your father's not well" he was going. And the letter didn't actually say a lot. It was left . . . I got upset and whatever, and the first thing that came into my head was that it is Hodgkinson's Disease, you know, and sort of I tried to find out about it. Just because they sound a bit similar with the two H's, you know. And the next thing you know I am straight on the phone to Dad.

MK: So the letter didn't actually say Huntington's?

ID: It said Huntington's but it didn't actually say [it was the case that Bruno had it] . . . It just sort of said, "you need to tell the children of this disease".

MK: And the letter was written to Susie? Saying it was her responsibility to tell?

ID: *Addressed* [emphasis] to Susie. It didn't say that he felt that it was better that she would have to tell us. Susie read it first I suppose. We both read it. I think I must have read it over his [Bruno's] shoulder, I can't really remember. You remember the aftermath of sort of picking up the phone and phoning him [Oliver] and saying, "Well look, what is this disease?" And sort of him going "Calm down, you need to go to your doctor". So the first thing I did was get on the phone, because we had a very good paediatrician for the Down's at the hospital for Stefan, and we explained it all to him. And he said you obviously need to talk about it. "Come and see me this afternoon". So that is what we did and he basically in a very simple way explained what it was and arranged for us to go for some genetic counselling.

Faced with the prospect of caring for a dying husband and looking after two young children, one of whom is affected with Down's syndrome, the worst thing of all, Isobel explains, is living with the burdensome knowledge that one or both of her children may have inherited the Huntington's gene. Though not herself genetically predisposed to HD, Isobel embodies the 'riskiness' of a pre-symptomatic person caught between the temporality of diagnosis and prognosis. Whilst 'preparing' herself for the eventuality of Bruno's predictable decline, she inhabits a chronic 'death-space' (see Chapter 3) of uncertainty and ambivalence in which she is obligated not simply as a Huntington's in-marrying wife but as the living testimony to Bruno's progressive decomposition. How in later years will she tell her children about their father? And what will they, in turn, decide to pass on to others as 'ethical' memory, as their version of genetically reconstructed knowledge? Will they transmit 'an Oliver'? What does Isobel need to do to avert this? This morally loaded pre-emptive death space also evokes the same strain of 'riskiness' that Daisy Opie acted to avert by deflecting the news of her positive test result from her father. Unlike Jack, Isobel however *does* carry the foreknowledge her children might turn into the shadow of her spouse. Remember that Jack's greatest fear was that Daisy and Liz would find themselves transformed physically into the eventuality of their mother's illness and thus become 'like' Mary. We may say that Isobel and Daisy, as agents embodying the effects of knowledge transmission and revelation come to be 'related' as partners in a dynamic social genealogy of non-disclosure, misinformation and partial 'un-truths'. As we shall go on to see, the ways each of these relatives choose to activate kin as relations of moral knowledge remains variably discrepant and unpredictable. This observation alone already confounds traditional biomedical presumptions since it shows that personal genetic information cannot be simply isomorphic with claims to individual autonomy. This, by implication, raises the question of the extent to which 'the right not to know' can be adequately conceptualised in genethics discourse as problems defined solely in terms of breaches of personal confidentiality and unsolicited disclosure. I turn now for comparative relief to the work of three British medical anthropologists whose writing has touched on the themes of embodiment and moral knowledge in ways that are pertinent to the present discussion on genetic knowledge and the ethics of disclosure.

Rethinking the importance of knowing about not knowing

In a paper on contemporary Hausa medical culture entitled 'The importance of knowing about not knowing', Murray Last (1981) considers why Nigerian patients and practitioners from the Malumfashi area (Kaduna state) display a strong indifference towards sources of health information. The attitude of not knowing or not caring to know about the causes, manifestations and treatment of various illnesses is not simply a matter of wilful ignorance but is part of the institutionalisation of health. Institutional power is shaped largely in this setting by the non-legitimisation of alternative discourses of health expertise by state authorities and has led to a potent mix of medical anarchism and pluralism. In brief, Last describes how Hausa medicine historically encompasses a diverse medical culture that originates, in part, from the large influx of immigrant populations to the area since the 1890s and during the territorial expansions of colonial rule from the early 1900s. During this time the traditional medicines of the Muslim Maguzawa, the herbal remedies of Islamic medicine and the practices of Western (hospital) medicine began to comprise overlapping areas of specialisation. The mix of knowledge expertise continues today but it has become increasingly difficult to preserve former professional distinctions, say, between the remedies dispensed by a *boka* (healer) and the spirit possession rituals performed by a *mai Danko* (master of the fearsome spirit of Danko). And as the range of traditional healers does not adhere to a single consistent theory,[9] traditional medicine is too diffuse and seemingly anarchic to be monopolised. Unable to form exclusive professional groups, healers become 'un-systematised' and people's health-seeking behaviour conforms rather to an ethno-ecological folk belief theory that equates appropriate treatments with the place from which the patient is known to have originated.

One of the noteworthy observations in this analysis concerns the extent to which medical indifference, including the non-revelation of sources of knowledge and secrecy about ailments, produces a climate of disinformation amongst patients and their kin. Last remarks that this culture of non-knowledge also elides distinctions between lay and expert claims to information with the effect that '. . . people really do *not* know, truly "don't know" through a combination of secrecy, uncertainty and scepticism' (Last 1981:391, emphasis original). One might add that such pervasive institutionalisation of secrecy appears to invalidate separate orders or domains of health knowledge and represents a kind of 'total social fact', rather than any kind of intrinsic order of 'ignorance' or 'irrational' knowledge. In highlighting the social dimensions between local medical practice and non-knowledge, Last concludes by posing a complex theoretical question about the analytical salience of the etic construct of medical pluralism. Might not medical pluralism be an exaggerated, conceptually overburdened concept if what seems 'to the outsider a Babel of different medical ideas [is] to the insider an adequately homogenous means of coping with illness in all its forms' (*ibid*:391). There is one lingering clue as to why these means of coping may not be as homogenous after all. Not-knowing is also symptomatic of the recent decline of 'clan secrets' and the related breakdown in Hausa culture of lineages and wider kin groupings. In recent times, people have been turning towards a more 'personal' form of secret knowledge, partly in response to the fear of witchcraft accusations and as a cultural means to deflect personalised blame for misfortune events. The popularity of more 'personal secrets' appears also to go hand in hand, Last observes, with the increasing individualisation of medicine and the moral expectation that persons will have to rely to a far greater extent in the future on their own medical defences. This is not too unlike the encroaching ideology of geneticisation whereby appropriately informed genetic citizens are fashioned into moral subjects by virtue of the expectation that one need take active responsibility for one's health status.

We can see Last's analysis of 'the importance of knowing about not knowing' sets up ethno-ethical relief for the critical study of how knowledge circulates as social value and a source of ambivalence within competing medical (sub) systems. More broadly still, it shows how medicines in non-technologically advanced contexts may likewise engender social value for the (non)information they generate and in terms that appear negligible to a 'rights' based discourse.

Where Last's discussion focuses mainly on macro-structural forces and the wider play of institutional power, Gilbert Lewis (1995) and Cecilia McCallum (1996) consider the relationship between moral knowledge and social agency, in particular bringing to the fore questions of temporality and illness belief. Lewis has made repeated visits to small isolated villages inhabited by the Gnau people of West Sepik province, Papua New Guinea and much like Susan Reynolds Whyte's work on the Bunyole of Eastern Uganda (see Chapter 3), he argues that Gnau diagnoses are applied to syndromes of circumstance rather than syndromes of clinical symptoms and signs. A key component of such diagnoses lies in the understanding of illness as moral events intricately related to the *past actions* and beliefs of agents. Hence the Gnau come to understand how social relations may be 'revealed by illness' due to, say, stolen food that has been wrongly eaten, or the way particular crops have been tended, or the watchful actions of spirits. Since danger may be recognisable only retrospectively because it has been 'shown up' by the illness, the events surrounding the time of illness exemplify a certain moral register that 'may put beliefs at stake, recall actions for questioning' (Lewis 1995:175). But these illness events are not simply circumstantial episodes. Lewis stresses it is how recent events come to be narrated through talk – crucially what evidence is left unsaid – that explains how causes may be deduced, and how listeners will be alerted to the moral significance of certain past events as actions implicating illness trajectories.

This temporally embedded chain of conjunctive associations features still more strongly in Cecilia McCallum's (1996, 2001) analysis of the links between health and embodied agency as perceived by the Cashinahua (Huni Kuin) peoples from the Brazilian-Peruvian borderlands in Amazonia. McCallum argues that the inextricable interrelations between health, knowledge and social identity set up an 'ethno-epistemology' of the Cashinahua body. In this account, the interconnected processes whereby the Cashinahua 'person' is (embodied as) an accumulation of social knowledge are traced as events that can be located in the temporality of the acting body. For the Cashinahua, the body is a social entity that is being continuously 'grown' out of the environment by the agency of others. The transformative processes that constitute the 'making grow' (*yume wa-*) of the 'Cashinahua body' over the course of a person's life depend on knowledge that others have acquired, and thus implicate these acts of (bodily) growth in social and moral questions about kinship, gender and ethics. Social action takes the form of 'the exteriorisation of knowledge' since 'social process constantly hinges on people who know making the knowing bodies of others' (MacCallum 1996:357, 364). Since in this view the very concept of health is understood as a combination of accumulated knowledge and the ability to act on it socially, illness, by implication, can be understood as '*a disturbance in the body's capacity to know*' (McCallum 1996, emphasis original). So, in this particular example the importance of knowing about not knowing turns out to be as vital as constitutional substance itself: it is literally a matter of survival and well being.

Now Western medical taxonomy, unlike the classificatory systems of the indigenous Cashinahua, does not categorise an ill body as one that no longer knows, except – somewhat dubiously – in cases of extreme mental illness and pathological disturbance. Nor do British people and other English-speaking Westerners *routinely* associate healing treatments as actions focused specifi-cally on the restoration of a person's *capacity to know*. What to the Westerner would be meaningful as acts of 'socialisation' commencing with the child infant – and the attendant notion of the social self constructed upon a biolog-ical strata of 'natural' being – entails for non-Europeans the incessant corpo-real integration of different kinds of knowledge acquired over time as certain 'growth'. Knowledge may even be localised in some cases in different body parts. For the Cashinahua, speech can act upon the bodies of listeners to create a moral disposition for sociability and similar effects can be induced through the workings of so-called ear knowledge, skin knowledge, hand knowledge or eye knowledge.[10] Despite these clear inter-regional differences in conceptions of personhood, there may, however, be subtle similarities at work that render the non-knowing bodies of my Huntington's families and others more akin with the Cashinahua 'knowing' bodies than would at first be suspected. There is, after all, a sense in which Isobel and Daisy's narratives are stories that talk of ill bodies and persons as social entities that no longer know. When Daisy for instance says she acts to shield her father 'in the same way that he withheld information from me about mother', these actions of mutual shielding are not totally unlike the 'protective' organs of Cashinahua body knowledge.

Foreknowledge and the liabilities of veracity

'Drawing the line at telling': Isobel's dilemmas

Bok's (1982) observation that some secrets exercise paradoxical power by simultaneously protecting and harming persons are contradictions Isobel attempts to negotiate less by recourse to a fixed ethical principle or abstract bioethical guideline than by living the everyday. Deciding when a lie is not a lie and when the inauguration of an 'untruth' might be legitimate is an ethical 'intensity' she works out as emergent practice. In thinking about the best way to transmit knowledge about Bruno's illness to Stefan, aged 7, and Louisa, aged 5, Isobel talks about how best to negotiate the moral boundaries between truth and untruth. She evokes the creative processes of muddling through and getting by.

ID: . . . my immediate concern is what effect giving a child of five the knowledge that one day he may have the same . . . And that is where I have come unstuck because it seems such a harsh thing to give a five-year-old that knowledge. And Louisa is a worrier and she will go away and be worried about it. So the next question is . . . she knows what hereditary means and we have used the word hereditary so I don't think it is going to be in the next year, but it could be that question is going to be asked . . . Yes, it will be hard dealing with that knowledge . . . Trying to teach them not to tell lies, and drawing the line at telling [them that] they may develop the disease . . .

MK: How did you explain 'hereditary' to her?

ID: I did say that that means that Daddy's Daddy had it. Then Daddy got it. That is hereditary and . . . I can't remember, it was just a quick and straightforward thing which she seemed happy with. But afterwards I thought, well, is she going to come back and ask: "Does that mean that I will get it too?" Which she didn't and hasn't. But she can think about things for months, and she has come back with a question, so I think it will come.

Some years ago the feminist sociologist Barbara Katz Rothman (1986) described the uncertain birth predicaments experienced by a diverse group of North American mothers undergoing prenatal testing. She suggested these conceptions were, in her words, 'tentative pregnancies'. Amniocentesis and other tests made the mother-to-be into a person who tended to withhold establishing strong gestational connections with her growing embryo until such time as the baby could be confirmed medically as a viable lifeform (cf. Rapp 1999;

Browner and Press 1995). Similarly, one may say that for a large number of families affected by certain hereditary illnesses, people establish relatedness through the uncertainties that mark out a 'tentative genealogy'. Such uncertainties show up clearly against the experiential backdrop of predictive genetic testing outcomes – outcomes that are played out as various kinship scenarios concerning the intra and inter-generational exchange of genetic knowledge between 'at risk' persons or HD affected kin.

For the Daley family, the fundamental meaning of heredity has become interlaced with how, and crucially how much, genetic knowledge Isobel thinks she should reveal over time to her young potentially 'at risk' children. In such cases, heredity is not simply about the objective existence of a known and specific biological tie, nor is it evidence of what can count as a past genetic transmission. It is, rather, about how the cultural recognition of a particular genetic tie implicates a particular 'genealogical ethics' as tentative. What Isobel, and numerous other similarly placed parents talk about, is how they decide to evoke certain genetic knowledge as local moralities of (non) disclosure. It is these decisions, grounded in the deeply situational and context-laden nature of everyday social intercourse, as opposed to the clinical protocol of biomedical procedure and bioethical 'first principles', that give moral shape and affective meaning to these embodied forms of moral knowledge. During our conversation, Isobel indicates she is aware that it is not just what she says to Louise (and Stefan) that matters, but how she decides to tell knowledge as 'truth' to her. Her tactics of disclosure emerge as highly contextual moral action that takes account of several considerations: the questions her daughter asks, her general emotional capacity at any particular time, and how much information she thinks she can deal with on that given day. This creative, richly textured morality unfolds as a pragmatic kind of 'drip-by-drip' approach to truth-telling that is sensitive to the timing of disclosure and to how knowledge is conveyed, rather than to any pure ontological sense of unmediated substance.[11] An ethics of disclosure, in other words, works itself out over time as a series of staggered revelations.

Understanding how different actors negotiate or muddle through a genealogical ethics in such contexts often involves much reconstructive work for the social scientist as bioethnographer. Often such critical bioethnographies will be of a speculative nature with moments of 'revelation' only coming to light as inconspicuous 'non-evidence' from the multiple perspective of various standpoints. Isobel's comments about her in-laws are narrated for instance from her singular viewpoint since it had proved impossible for me to arrange to meet Oliver himself, nor to establish contact with Pete and Susie. Though Bruno was happy to meet and we did attempt to converse, there were understandable constraints to his participation. Can we still see the larger picture though?

Oliver's own failing health, having been revealed by the retrospective and hypothetical speculations he had pieced together about his late father's illness, is
transformed into posthumous knowledge that 'travels' to his children (Bruno
and Diana) and grandchildren as mediated relatedness. It is through Susie and
Pete that Isobel and Bruno learn about Oliver, but it is also likely that Oliver's
search through his late father's papers was initiated by questions he would
have encountered at the genetic clinic about his medical genealogy. 'Is there
any hereditary illness in the family?' 'What did your father die of?' Oliver's
letter writing evolves in all likelihood from certain 'pressures' or advice he
receives from the counsellors about the need to 'stop' the disease in its tracks
(see Chapter 5). Certainly one may conjecture that Oliver would have been
'guided' by the clinic to get in touch with his estranged family in accordance
with their 'best interests'. Working out the best interests of others is of course a
purely abstract speculation on the part of the counsellors who can know nothing
more about Bruno and Isobel than what Oliver will have sketched in for them,
most probably during a half hour's counselling appointment. Similarly, it is
also probable that Oliver was 'forewarned' about the machinery of unsolicited
disclosure that could swing into action should he refuse himself to re-establish
contact voluntarily. As an exercise in critical narratology, we can join up these
loose unarticulated threads at the point where Isobel first knows she has become
'revealed by [another's] illness' (cf. Lewis 1995; also Armstrong *et al.* 1998).
But as I have been stressing, there are several layers to the form such revelation takes. A key moment is clearly the concession that Isobel may well have
reconsidered the viability of her future procreative relation to Bruno had Oliver
acted upon his worst suspicions about his father's hereditary past and shared
the 'truth' with others far sooner. Another temporal staging of this 'revelation' occurs when Isobel painfully recalls how, looking back on events, there
were indeed signs that not all was well physically with her father-in-law on the
day of her wedding.

What then are the revealing gaps? Certainly we can say that we do not
know for how long Oliver was pre-symptomatic and then mildly symptomatic
before receiving his diagnosis and being recognised *by others* as unwell
(cf. the ethnographer's misrecognition and the case of Lucy Williams discussed
in Chapter 3). It is not even the case that the truth lies latent since we have not
been able to trace whether in fact Oliver perceived his accumulating knowledge
as a 'growth' that would necessarily implicate others over time as part of a
sociality of pre-emptive relatedness (cf. McCallum 1996). What Isobel omits
from her account is how Oliver's decision to delay disclosure may well have
reflected his own indecisive and uncertain knowledge about himself. It is quite
possible he had not wanted to alarm the family by giving them a 'false positive',

the harmful burden of indeterminate knowledge that may turn out to have no biological or social grounding. Whether or not this is the case, I simply draw attention to the way such a possibility appears to have been *written out* of the transmitted interfamilial record (cf. Bailey 1991). And yet, if my speculations hold ground, Oliver's 'untruth' is actually the very same dilemma facing both Isobel and Daisy in the present day as they struggle to find a suitable language in which to communicate with their young offspring the eventuality of predispositional personhood. Both women are reluctant to tell their children about the presence of the disease in the family unless they were already party to the unequivocal foreknowledge their children definitely *are* positive carriers. As Whyte (1997:215) notes of her Nyole informants: 'uncertainty is sometimes preferable to a certainty that is too painful. But uncertainty can also prove deadly for others' (see Chapter 3).

'Time will tell': Daisy's decisions

Much like Isobel, Daisy develops a pre-symptomatic strategy of being 'economical' with the truth and staggering the disclosure about her mother's illness and her own positive HD status. Fragments of knowledge are metered out over time in an unstructured and informal fashion to accommodate and respond to her children's intermittent enquiries. Ethical decisions about disclosure relate to the way her children are being cultivated as 'at risk' persons, a point to which we return in Chapter 6. Yet there is also a fair amount of pre-emptive planning for future action that is about making kinship in anticipation of Daisy's imminent illness.

DO: ... one of the things I wanted was that it was going to be open. I wanted the kids to grow up with like. . . . "Okay, we've got this thing in our family", and that's it, sort of thing. It's like "Yeah, okay, Nanny was ill and Mummy is a bit poorly". When they're older, I want that to happen. I don't want it to suddenly like "Sit down, I've got something to tell you". But, on the other hand, I didn't want to have to give them this information over the years if I didn't need to. I didn't want to, you know, if I was negative. And then they could go through life and not even think about it, you know. That was my main reason for going for the test, you see. I wanted to know so I knew whether they needed to know. So umm . . . time will tell, but there's never going to be a long major talk.

MK: Yes.

DO: And because Jamie's so worried about death at the moment after losing [my] Dad. I didn't want to say "Well, Mummy's going to get it and it's gradually going to get worse as she gets older and she's not going to get better from it". You know, so I left it at that. I thought well just wait for the next question. It didn't come luckily.

Both Isobel and Daisy's narratives point to some of the trying moral navigation work parents undertake as local negotiations of 'unsolicited disclosure'. We have seen that people's local appropriations of 'beneficence' and 'non-maleficence', in contrast to mainstream bioethics and formal principles, are not necessarily weighed up in a rational or self-maximising utilitarianism as competing 'virtues'. The ethnographic commentary shows rather how local understandings and values emerge from certain pragmatic subversions of 'the truth' that complicate the very authenticity of the designs of 'truth' itself. Unlike the authoritative channels of power through which most clinicians steer procedures of 'truth' telling, parents live in daily contact with the less predictable effects that anticipatory foreknowledge of the new genetic testing technology opens up. They are thus much more susceptible to the paradoxes such experiential knowledge brings, yet ironically have much more specialist knowledge at their disposal about the difficulties divergent kin encounter in reaching any kind of ethical resolution to the dilemmas they continuously live with.

   The previous sections have highlighted several points about the intricacies of kinship talk and its relation to family dilemmas and ethical decision-making concerning the new genetics. First we have been able to identify how the genethics discourse of information disclosure entails emergent moralities of kinship (non) disclosure. The view that genes are isomorphic with 'decoded' information that ought to be shared as well as the paradoxical prescriptivism of 'non-directed' counselling are both versions of 'truth' that are shown to be wanting. We considered how these kinship moralities more accurately negotiate a diverse 'family of untruths' as forms of complicity and non-knowledge exchanged over time, rather than sets of obligations or entitled rights in and over people as customarily defined by the complex of 'kinship' in social anthropology. We further explored how these 'untruths' can be shaded in as different ethical intensities and embodied in divergent ways as particular knowledge *flows*. These flows, as part of a complex relational ethics (see Chapters 5 and 6), necessarily challenge the sense in which the conventional bioethical register presumes that claims to 'the right to know' or even 'the right not to know' about genetic information can be advanced by autonomous self-regarding and self-unitary individuals. Further, ethnographic analysis of the ethics of kinship disclosure points to how there is nothing inherently predictable about the way people 'set apart' knowledge as the actions of discernment, and thus produce 'hidden' knowledge as the objectification of 'secrets'. I have argued instead that these moral genealogies are continuously active and 'under construction' as a living genealogical ethics. They are not static, frozen objectifications of an abstract or disembodied time-frame, but commentaries on the ongoing experiences and effects of 'prophetic genetics'. If these commentaries tell us about the embodied incorporation of predictive testing as rituals of experimental technology, such talk illuminates the difficult 'coming into being' of pre-symptomatic persons by filling in what one user group – in speaking of the unintended consequences of 'unsolicited disclosure' – has referred to as 'a leap in the dark'.[12]

PART III

Relational ethics in practice

5

Reproducing exclusion

In Chapter 4 we considered two substantive concerns informing an anthropological 'ethno-ethics' for the anticipatory study of probable life futures related to developments in predictive testing technologies. These are characterised by the dual attempt to (1) delineate kinship relations as changing techniques of heredity and moral genealogy; and (2) show how certain forms of relatedness are fundamentally at odds with the bioethical conception of individual autonomy that underpins the medicocentrism of 'rights'-based claims to knowledge. When the issues underscoring the 'right to know/right not to know' debates are transposed ethnographically to a microanalysis of real-time decision-making, we are able to see how the 'facts' of a genealogical ethics are built up over time as local moralities of information disclosure and non-disclosure. While family members must discriminate between genetic information that they think is good to know or make known, and knowledge that they think is 'bad' to tell and share with others, such attempts frequently entail unresolved processes of moral decision-making, both within and across the generations. As embodied experiences of moral reckoning, these genealogical knowledge dilemmas also implicate a myriad of interests and divergent claims beyond the life of any one person. Now these plural interests, and their activation by social agents in the experience of everyday genetics, require the conceptual modelling of a relational ethics in contradistinction to earlier evolution-based accounts of a so-called 'naturalistic ethics'.

We saw previously that a handful of earlier anthropological critiques of sociobiology in the 1970s had started to challenge the biological appropriation of 'culture' put forward by neo-Darwinian kin selection theory (see Chapter 2). The 'gene's eye perspective', synonymous with the view that it is not the survival of the individual organism that counts ultimately, but rather the survival of copies of the gene itself, remains today a popular belief among 'gene-selectionist' evolutionary theorists whose articulations, at worst, reproduce dangerous forms of biological essentialism. Rose and Rose (2000) take to task some of the most disturbing discourses to have surfaced in recent years in their critique of evolutionary psychology. The renewed turn to genes and genetics as *the* ideological basis for causal explanations of human behaviour (the belief in the existence of such things as 'gay genes', 'criminal genes', 'genes for drunkenness' and so on) is a modern manifestation of an older fundamentalism. Edward Wilson's 'naturalistic ethics', for example, in stressing the evolutionary basis of morality advocates the view that human morality may be embedded quite literally in our genes as 'the innate epigenetic rules of moral reasoning' (1998:283). This belief that moral value comprises an intrinsic part of our biological heritage derived originally from the nineteenth-century notion of an 'evolutionary ethics' as propounded by British philosopher and sociologist Herbert Spencer (who became famous for the neologism 'survival of the fittest'). It should not escape contemporary discussions of 'genetic altruism', particularly in relation to the ethics of gene banking, that evolutionary ethics was updated as William 'Bill' Hamilton's (1964, 1975) sociobiological thesis of 'inclusive fitness' and its purported linking together of morality and biology through the genetics of altruism.

To illustrate how kin selection entails complicated cultural processes between divergent moral agents (i.e. persons who believe themselves to be related through different degrees of genetic risk, genetic risk perception and experiences of predisposition), the next two chapters present four inter-related scenarios of kinship 'exclusion'. These detail the persistent, elusive and subtle interdependencies that may frame relatedness between social agents in these contexts, and thereby make known the rich tapestry of associations, emotion, vulnerability, uncertainty and ambivalence we can re-describe as a 'relational ethics'.

Testing kin loyalty

1. Loyal, loyalty; true to obligations of duty, love; faithful to plighted troth. 1604
2. Loyal, legalis, legal; of a child: legitimate
                    (*Oxford English Dictionary on Historical Principles*)

When one parent has been diagnosed and found positive, a particularly sensitive area is the relatedness between about-to-be-tested siblings. I would often hear brothers and sisters of different age groups talking about their perceptions of the projected effects of testing. Availing themselves of new genetic knowledge might alter, some said, what had formerly been assumed as a shared parity of doubt between them. Those who were living independently from one another and outside of the parental home would frequently confide in me, articulating such comments as: 'I'll talk to you [MK] and tell you my story, but please make sure you don't tell my result when you see my sister/brother'. Many would not be concerned simply to protect others in the family from disclosure of a bad result but would feel that good news too should have limited social circulation. This would apply both to those with happy news to divulge, and to those pre-symptomatic siblings 'in the know' who have been tested ahead of another sibling whose genetic status remains indeterminate. One positively tested woman I met at an HD social event said she would back away from her as yet untested sister were she to be confirmed with a negative status. 'We've been in the same boat', she went on to explain, 'had the same worry . . . [it's] pulling us together . . . [we're] now in the same boat . . . [in the] same situation'. Sometimes it is the sharing of uncertainty and the joint propensity to misfortune between siblings that comprises the primary kinship link, the strongest tie. In any case, concerns about the 'non-equivalence' of positive and negative test results between divergent kin carry considerable emotional resonance. The following two scenarios (involving the Kingston/Richardson and the Williams families) explore certain links between the acquisition of new genetic knowledge and the familial ruptures experienced by kin as they 'reproduce' in real-time forms of relatedness through a tactics of exclusion that variously 'turns against' their own.

"Outsiders within" – conflicts of interest and genetic escapees

Ann Kingston (née Thomason), late wife of Charles, spent the last ten years of her life in residential care. Except for their son Rex, the only sibling out of six not to be predisposed to HD, Charles has disowned himself as biological father of his other offspring. After each had decided to take the test, Charles declared he wanted nothing more to do with them. The family joke bitterly amongst themselves as they explain to me that the occasional card they receive from him at Christmas is signed Charles *Kingston*, a greeting they interpret as reminder their 'errant' bloodline is undeserving of the patrilineal family name. 'We're just Thomason', one of the Kingston sons keeps repeating. 'He sees as all as "Thomason"'. The Kingston siblings and their in-marrying affines are semi-skilled manual workers in their thirties and forties living with little disposable income. Though they are not particularly keen to talk to me about their planned financial futures, health insurance or the apportioning of their late mother's inheritance, a sense of family divisiveness comes across when they mention how infuriating it is to see their father pander 'all lovey dovey' to his girlfriend. She too, they explain, shuns the siblings but only has to 'lift a finger' to receive lavish gifts and other attentions from him. Much of this talk belies the conventional Euro-American understanding that 'blood' ties ought to implicate certain kinship obligations, and the associated disappointment that the consistency of 'blood' substance has been diluted over time by what the siblings see as displaced paternal loyalty.

But despair hit the family more shockingly when two of the six siblings took their lives a couple of years ago. Both of their in-marrying widows had young nursery school children at the time their husbands and fathers 'disappeared'. The remaining Kingston siblings feel traumatised and vulnerable. Besides Ben, a lorry driver who is single and to his knowledge fatherless, his two HD-affected sisters are responsible for the care of several teenage offspring. Elene and Pam, both positive, mother eleven children between them, not all of whom are genetically related as stepchildren. Rex, their non-HD affected brother, parents six children with his partner, Claire, and like himself two of his several nieces, Mabel and Nelly Richardson, are also 'in the clear' after going for pre-symptomatic testing to check a possible maternal transmission. (Elene, their mother, is now symptomatic). As they all explain, considerable conflicts of interest have surfaced across the family about the responsibilities of care giving, as well as wrangles between the affected and non-affected kin over the subject of who has 'got off' or escaped from the disease. Now, were one simply to read off objective kinship knowledge gleaned from the genealogical constructs of a medically annotated family tree – as drawn up by the nurse counsellors at the genetics clinic – the two sisters would be seen to occupy a structurally equivalent position with Uncle Rex. This threesome appear to be 'lucky', as they put it, in that they all have escaped what they know for others is a 'tragic' (the family's choice of word) genetic inheritance of compromised ill health. Nonetheless, their kinship talk is anchored in various idioms of misfortune, regret and divisiveness. They all say they feel like 'outsiders' within the family and talk of themselves as 'excluded' often referring to one another as 'the odd ones out'. Rex describes the kinship between himself and nieces Mabel and Nelly as

> a bond . . . [we're] bonded through exclusion . . . we're set apart from others, we're on our own, it's like everybody else on the outside looking in. [It's] just between us. . . . it's an uneven. . . . it will become harder as others become iller [sic] . . .

In the following excerpts, Rex and his nieces articulate an emergent kinship morality based on their self-identification as 'escapees' from a genetic future that has already destroyed the lives of (deceased uncles) Patrick and Arthur.

It is just there, a guilty feeling, all the time. There is never a day goes by when you don't think about it, when you don't feel bad about it in some way. I mean in a couple of years time, I am going to be the only one out of all of us who is still here . . . And then there's my sisters' kids. It is never ending. It feels as though we [Nelly and Mabel] are the odd ones out. I remember thinking after the test, for quite a while, I wished I had had a bad result, so you know I could be the same as the rest. I just wanted to be the same as everybody else. I didn't want to be the odd one out.

I thought if I get a good result, it would be like a bit weight off my shoulders. It would be a bit of freedom, basically a big weight off my shoulders, like a release. A bit more happiness, but it didn't work out as I thought it would at all. In fact I think it was worse after the test than it was before . . . (Rex)

Mabel explains how after a long period of doubt and much procrastination she finally arrived at the decision to get tested.

My boyfriend knew that I could not go on the way I was. Just not knowing. Whatever I decided to do, he backed me all the way. He knew that I was so unhappy. I was on anti depressants. I just could not cope with not knowing. So I convinced myself really that everything was, the rest of my life was going to be crap anyway, so I would not have anything to lose really.

But since taking the test her views have changed. Now she expresses concerns that her younger siblings who are not yet old enough to take the test should not follow her example. Since a future generation of 'at risk' persons is clearly emergent in this family, Mabel and Nelly speak not just for their siblings, but also implicitly for what they assume would constitute the future well being of several cousins.

MR: Yes, I have told them that I don't want them to [take the test], even though it can go either way. It still was the worst day of my life, and sometimes I wish I had never done it. I wish I hadn't. I was happier 18 months ago, more than I am now. I was. I just didn't think about it. Put it to the back of my mind and didn't think about it. And now it is there all the time.

MK: So you do actually in a sense regret the knowledge that you have?

MR: Because of everybody else, because of what is happening to everybody else. I mean, I feel that I don't even belong here. When I look at Ben and then I think "why am I here?" And I think, "that is what they are thinking". I think that is what they are thinking: that I should not be here.

I have got a good result. I should be off enjoying life. And we are all talking about Huntington's and I am not even going to get it. And they are there . . . It has slightly changed, it is not in the same way obviously, but it is never going to go away, anyway, just because I have done that. It is never going to go away. And instead of the worry about yourself

eating you up all of the time, it is the worry of everybody else. And the
guilt that it is not going to get any better as well.

I know it sounds stupid, but I said to my sister about a week after I
had my test, you know – she put off having her results for a while. And
I remember going around to her house for a coffee about a week after.
I was just really down and was having a bad day. And she said to me,
"What is wrong with you?" "You have just had the all clear, you should
be on cloud nine". "I don't feel like that at all", I said. And she said, "I
think that is really selfish. I would do anything to have that result". And
it threw me. That that was what she thought.

When I interview Nelly, Mabel's sister, the sentiments sound familiar though
her situation is somewhat different: a recent divorcee in her early twenties
she now carries the responsibilities of a full-time single mother to two young
children. She talks about the open resentment directed to her by one of her
maternal aunts and the awkwardness generated by her newly acquired genetic
knowledge which she took care not to disclose directly herself.

NR: I thought I would be happy about a good result, but I didn't really. I just
       felt guilty. And I saw our Sally after and she said [on behalf of my aunt],
       "That is not fair you got a good result and I got a bad one". Which made
       me a lot worse, because I felt bad enough already.
MK: Can you remember what she said exactly?
NR: I did not actually tell her myself that I had got a good result. Someone
       had told her and she came in to me where I was, and said, "I have heard
       about you going and getting your test results, and I don't think that is
       fair, I think I should have it". And I said, "I feel guilty enough already"
       and later on she said sorry about it, but I do feel funny around her now.

These points of view serve to show how conflicts of difference between the
Kingston/Richardson kin have become demarcated along clearly 'genetic' lines.
The families appear to extend into a kinship-fractured divisiveness between
those who are 'positive' and those who are 'negative'. Yet even those who have
tested negative do not feel themselves to be free of the disease since the affliction
of disease becomes everybody's disorder and heredity engenders far more than
simply the lineal inheritance of 'risky' genes. It is not just the illness itself but
the knowledge of it that gets reproduced between kin. The foreknowledge that a
tentative genealogy is shared and implicates a common future is knowledge that
affects everyone. As Mabel says 'It's never going to go away – we're all in it'.[1]
If others see it as the good fortune of Mabel, Nelly and Rex to be excluded as

genetic 'escapees', Rex turns this around with the dramatic statement 'I wished I had had a bad result, so you know I could be the same as the rest'. The wish to be able to undo certain knowledge and reverse his genetic inheritance is a refusal to equate 'good' genes as enough of a criterion to stop the line of biological transmission. That kin do not divide themselves simply into mutually exclusive bounded groups according to their genetic prognosis is something that Claire, Rex's partner, wants to make clear. When she talks implicitly of an intra-familial ranking and evaluation of social suffering that makes events and relations other than what they seem (cf. 'the liabilities of veracity' explored in Chapter 4), her intervention has the effect of acknowledging Rex's involvement in the family's future suffering. For her, biology is simply an inaccurate marker of a person's social predicament. This turning away from genetics as an explanatory idiom for the family's misfortune – reasoned here as a form of 'de-geneticisation' – is inflected with the same sense of anticipatory foreknowledge that disturbs Mabel and Nelly:

Claire: I think in one way, yes, you know, you get a good result because there are kids involved as well. But there are times when you think, they [the rest of the family] think because Rex has got a good result, well he has got nothing to worry about, you know. He gets very very depressed about the rest of the family. Still losing brothers and sisters . . . it is still harder for the living that carry on living than what it is you know for the ones that are here. And he is the one that has got to see them all slowly go, and then as more family go through the same, *so in some respects I think that Rex has got it harder* (emphasis added) But because he has got a good result, the others see it as he is alright.

The Kingston family are testimony to the making of 'mixed narratives' within particular familial groupings – on the one hand, certain kin appear to reinforce the primacy of a genetic way of thinking, whilst a number of implicated kin within the same family unit instigate a differently conceived 'de-geneticisation' of knowledge. At the same time, these narratives illustrate how people acquire an inchoate vocabulary for the documentation of a past subjunctive. Predictive genetic testing technology sets up the expectation that kin should be able to talk about certain (non) events that *could have* come to pass.

Sometimes genetic 'escapees' may forego the knowledge that they could have been adversely affected yet nonetheless feel in some sense compromised. An example would be children whose 'at risk' parent withholds knowledge of a clear test result before introducing the topic of HD to explain what otherwise could have affected the family. After receiving Dylan's negative genetic test, the Jeffrys find it difficult to break the 'good' news to their children that they are no longer at risk of hereditary complications for HD (see Chapter 3). Parents Dylan and Ruth try to tell Michael, aged 18, and Sandy, aged 10, that a former uncertainty has been removed from their lives. But, as they say, it is hard to know how to formulate and explain quite what it now means to know one is no longer at a possible risk.

> We told the children then everything. It was a bit difficult for them to comprehend at that moment. It took a lot of conversations over the ensuing weeks for them really to understand. They were resentful at first that they had been excluded from knowing what was going on – but we still feel that we made the right decision for us not to tell them at that time. I think they felt that we didn't trust them but it's not as simple as that.
>
> Again I had to act as mediator. I really had to impress on Michael that if he really thought about it that Dylan was extremely brave in making the decision to get tested as he did. If the result had been positive then life would have become very difficult – it was very difficult to deal with before, a positive result would have made it impossible.
>
> *(Ruth Jeffrys)*

Unlike their parents, the Jeffrys children have not embodied over time the knowledge of what the future would hold had they been genetically predisposed. For them, simply finding out 'what might have been' is an abstract knowledge and of a quite different order to the 'revelations' retrospectively acquired by, say, someone like Isobel Daley (see Chapter 4) in her newly instigated role as in-marrying wife and carer to Bruno. This kind of subjunctive talk by parents, characterised especially by the difficulty of broaching the subject of prophetic genetics with offspring – even in cases when a genetic risk has been allayed – is not unlike the kind of worries siblings express concerning the preservation of a shared parity of intentional unknowingness. Both scenarios evoke the demands of grappling with the effects of indeterminate knowledge as unexpected alliances. These scenarios show in addition how genetic discrimination may be exercised within families as subtle forms of pressure and difference. Thus bio-surveillance may work discreetly inside of families as well as without. And as the monitoring of predispositional 'truths' goes beyond external bodies and public agencies, so family members re-negotiate their 'place' within existing kinship structures. Such a privatisation of genetic discrimination gives a different inflection to the commodification of genetic information that is publicly owned as DNA 'state' secrets and then 'sold off' to private drug companies.[2] One new genealogical fact therefore emerges: inside families, people are already busy 'privatising' their DNA and re-negotiating in the process the meaning they attach to heredity and to ties of relatedness.

Blood may be thicker than water, but genes don't only cross sexes ...

Learning to live with the news occasioned by each family member's test result, Lucy (who has tested positive, see Chapter 3) has been speculating what would have happened had her husband, Rupert, turned out to be the only unaffected person. Had both their sons Laurie and Hanno also tested positive, this would have introduced a non-equivalence of kin relations, or, as she puts it 'there would have been three persons against one'. The prospect of Rupert's sole exclusion from HD had unsettled her since she envisioned the possibility as the beginning of the un-making of affinal relatedness. In this 'three versus one' scenario, she and Rupert would be more likely to bifurcate into unlinked pairs, she explains, to 'de-couple' from each other as conjugal partners. This is a rather startling revelation about the value placed on genes as biological markers of kinship and cultural differentiation. Lucy appears to be privileging the biological and genetic factor of common linkage over associations that have been built up over time between kin as meaningful relations. However, because she anticipates – correctly as it turns out – which of her sons is likely to test positive, she also imagines the deepening of a split dividing Laurie and herself 'against' Hanno and Rupert. As a new 'genealogical fact', this remixing of kinship loyalties has the remedial feature of 'balancing up' what would otherwise connote an uneven distribution of illness misfortune within the family. I should stress that this is a condensed summary of Lucy's own interpretation of her worst fears.

"Everyone is a master of something": The Kung Fu dispute

As was made evident to me through the family's retrospective narration of a domestic row, a sense of relationality comprised out of persons who can change 'sides' and shift alliances did in fact materialise in real-time. A heated argument had taken place one evening on the subject of authoritative knowledge claims. The two brothers had literally come to blows over who and how others can claim to own particular knowledge and expertise. Seen as competing concepts of mastery and physical process, foreknowledge becomes the idiom through which the siblings compete to express their alternate belief in social engagement as democratisation. Different things, they claim, can be done to and with the power of knowledge. The different versions of the dispute presented here indicate how the abstract power of genetic science to 'determine' a person's physical constitution is deflected by ex-testees into a non-genetic domain, contrary in fact to Lucy's feared anticipations.

Lucy's account:

> I was worried that we had become a family divided into two. "The two that have" and "the two that haven't". Or that we would be three that had it, and then there'd be Rupert as the odd one out. And that was my biggest fear. And then I thought afterwards, that it would be Rupert and Hanno that would be separate – there would be those two and then us two. But in fact what happened was what none of us had expected. You see we had a huge argument. It was an argument against. It was Hanno and I against Laurie. Or Laurie against Hanno and I.
>
> We had this argument about how to attain enlightenment and Hanno said he would like to find some master person, you know, and learn to be a great karate master. But it was just said in kind of . . . just as part of a conversation. Not that he was going off to be Bruce Lee or something! Well this was something that just flipped Laurie and he got really angry about it. This was really massive for him how stupid this was. And I then sided with Hanno and said, "That is not so stupid". And I remember thinking this is a silly argument. But Laurie took it to huge lengths to the point when he picked up a chair and said, "I will show you". And he was going to bash this over Hanno's head. It was that bad. And then we pushed him out of the door and he virtually started to break the door down, and was starting to smash things in the hall. I screamed for Rupert to get Laurie because we were scared. And then Laurie had got out of the house, and then Rupert went off with him and later Rupert came back and said we had wound Laurie up and sided with Laurie. It was very trivial and got very violent, you know, and violence is something that is new to our family, you know. We're like '60's "Love and peace, hey man", you know. It's just horrible.

Laurie's account:

> . . . my mother and I talk about it more now because it is a separate thing from my father and brother. There is this kind of divide almost. But it is not a large divide. It is almost like everyone has got their little place now. It is a strange feeling at times . . .
>
> . . . there is a definite change. How I would put that into words, I don't know? But, I mean, obviously there is a change because beforehand we were both brothers at risk, so neither of us knew. Neither did my parents know. . . .
>
> . . . At times I know it is stupid and I know it is completely wrong, and don't ask me how I know, but sometimes I feel like my father is treating my brother slightly differently to me. But I know that that is wrong because he is not. It is just suddenly my reaction to it all which is not . . . Which I know is totally wrong. Because I then think about it, and it is not right. It is just me. Everything is totally fine. I mean there is no . . . we are not treating each other any different because we are all educated, we all talk about it. A lot of families don't talk about it. Therefore they

end up treating each other differently because they don't share what they are feeling, and I am now more open to share more of what I am feeling, you see. More so now that I know that I have been tested positive, than I did before . . . .

. . . but I have a couple of times, I have had an argument with my mother and brother, and well, I completely flipped, smashed a few things to bits, . . . I literally cut my hand to shreds smashing the door in . . . and just left the place. And of course my father then came to my aid, and . . . you know he walked with me, chilled me out, and sorted it out. And basically, suddenly my mother and brother were now against my father and me, and we were against them. And suddenly that was a divide and I thought that was strange because it was like my father is supposed to be the carer for my mother, yet he was on my side. And my brother was supposed to be . . . I was supposed to be more on the side of my mother because we were both the ones with the gene. Yet Hanno was with her so that was a very odd situation, and it was cleared in a couple of days. We all chilled out and got back to normal, yeah.

Hanno's account:

I mean I can put that down to me and my brother really . . . Yes, it ended up in an argument. I was talking about something like kung fu lessons or something to have more inner peace. To be more aware of your body because we are all into this aikido thing and we were exercising a lot . . . . And I was mentioning about these kung fu lessons, and it was basically a conversation. And my brother's opinion was that you don't really need to do that. If you want to do that, you do it yourself. There is no difference. And I was saying "No you need to get taught by a master" and he went ballistic and said, "What constitutes a master?" you know. "Who says that person is a master? Master of what?" he was going. "I am a vegan. I am a master of veganism" he was saying. And I then said "No you're not." And he said, "Well, why am I not?" "You're just not," I said. He then went that he might not have a certificate to say I am a master of veganism, but he has done it all his life for twenty-four years so he's therefore a master compared to that guy walking down the street. Basically you can do it yourself. It is like "You can read a book and become educated" he was saying.

Laurie (continuing):

Then we came to HD and I was saying, "look, I know more than my family doctor about HD" Why? Have I done any lessons? No, I just learned myself. I read books. I go on the Internet. I read books. I talk to people who have experienced it. People who have lost their whole family to it. I now know more than my doctor, right? I can now class myself – not as a "master" – but maybe someone who is on their way to becoming a master. But, I *am* a master of veganism! [laughing] Fair enough, everyone is a master of something, right? Whether it is sitting in front of the telly and being a blob, you know what I mean? Everyone is a master of something. So, it was all this thing and it just got into this complete row . . . and I ended up saying that he was being totally ignorant and not allowing me to finish what I was saying and talking over what I was saying. I ended up saying that I was going to wrap the chair around his head basically . . . and he grabbed the chair before I did and raised it and I just ploughed straight into him. Of course my mother got between us. I ended up leaving the room and slammed the door after me. That is why I tried to beat the whole thing down with my fists – did myself damage in the end.

Rupert's account:

Well I didn't know whether I was going to be looking after three people, two people or one person. I now know there are two people I am going to be looking after. My wife Lucy and Laurie. It is better now that I know. It was a silly argument but helpful too. . . . I heard it from upstairs and came and said, "what the hell is going on?" . . .

. . . So yes, I mean I took Laurie's side inasmuch as I knew, well, my opinion was that you shouldn't, you know, provoke . . . My feeling was that Lucy and Hanno could have calmed the situation if they wanted to, and that two against one wasn't fair. That was the thing. They knew Laurie was going to flip. They knew if they kept persevering that he was going to flip . . . Going on and on and they just would not stop. And he just freaked because it was the two of them and they could have just stopped and said, "calm down for a moment". It was almost like they wanted to prove something and Laurie wanted to prove something. It just got out of hand, but as I said this is rare. It is a very rare thing 'cos we are an extremely close family.

A clinician reading these extracts may wish to point out that in some cases a tendency towards aggression and physical violence is part of the symptomatology of HD. Such biological extrapolations would tell only a fraction of the story however. Nor can processes of moral reasoning be attributed simply to one's genes. Much of the content of the dispute itself may be trivial but this does not detract from the fact that it is the process of conflict rather than any innate biological substance that mediates what counts as significant relations between the 'sidedness' of pre-symptomatic and non-affected kin. Through its comic-tragic resolution, kinship is seen to transmute into a contextual relational ethics for the intra-familial 'regulation' of appropriate flows of relatedness. Whilst Laurie's after-the-event verdict is that 'it is almost like everyone has got their little place now', it is actually in the narrating of the argument that Lucy and Laurie firm up how their shifting kin allegiances came to be worked out as non-genetically based relational configurations. Through his open support for son Laurie, father Rupert 'crosses over' what was formerly imagined to represent a line of genetic difference. He thereby 'mixes' together those Williams kin who are known to be HD-affected with those who are not. As a re-constituted moral network of affective relations, family members each develop their own discourse of skilled expertise that situates new genetic knowledge in extra-medical terms, whether through idioms of sport, fitness regimes, diet, clarity of vision or personal training.

Discussion: refiguring heredity as social anatomies of interdependence

The aforementioned family dispute and previous examples from Chapters 3 and 4 have illustrated how present and future forms of pre-emptive social exclusion require a more detailed understanding of 'new heredity' practices. A key conceptual feature of a relational ethics is its material grounding in what may be termed 'social anatomies of interdependence'.

The term 'social anatomy of interdependence' is modified here from anthropologist Jane Monnig Atkinson's notion of an 'anatomy of dependence' to describe the vital illness interventions of Wana shamans (Central Sulawesi, Indonesia) in the prevention and restoration of patients' good health (Atkinson 1989:102–19). Atkinson's study of Wana secret knowledge is derived in part from a detailed textual analysis of the songs recited during the healing ritual known as the 'potudu', a variant of the dramatic mabolong performances. Analysing the oratorical content of these performances, Atkinson suggests it is possible for the Wana to distinguish between the expert knowledge of 'verbal magic' (names and spells) and the material magic (the technical applications of medicine). Verbal magic is said to activate exclusive and 'hidden' knowledge that is skilfully accessed by the shaman through the special partnership cultivated with spirit familiars – where the structure of the non-visible as exclusive knowledge for interpretation by the few is analogous to the operations of Western secular 'science'.[3] Material magic, on the other hand, being substances of the everyday world, entails the simple application of medicines and basic spells for the treatment of overt symptoms, as opposed to unseen causes. Medicines, as one local informant reports, are unlike indigenous 'science': they are 'simply a technique' (*ojo salaak*) (*ibid*:75).

In this folk schemata of an indigenous science-technology split, expert knowledge and prosaic technology are valued as separate operations though we cannot necessarily overlay the ethnocentrism enjoining the distinction between 'fact' and 'value' upon the alternate systems of 'verbal' and 'material' magic. For many societies, the Wana being no exception, shamanic intervention is predicated on the therapeutic endeavours of journeying shamans whose efficacy depends on the extra-corporeal manipulations and transfers of their clients extracted or 'lost' body parts.[4] The potential for bodily modification is perceived to be part of a healing geography, part cognitive, part emotional, that requires the protracted mapping between the patient's inner anatomy and the geography of the cosmos. On the therapeutic journey of helper spirits to relieve a Cuna Indian woman's labour pains and assist with childbirth induction, Lévi-Strauss (1963:186–205) once described how the shamanic practices of Panamanian

Indians entail the healer's expedition into the womb. Vitebsky (1995:158), paraphrasing Lévi-Strauss, notes how once inside the patient's vagina 'their itinerary moves across a landscape which is both the internal anatomy of a living body and an emotional geography of the psyche which inhabits it'. As for local registers of morality, these implicitly justify the counter-invasions of spatialised modalities of the 'translocating' shaman. Wana shamans, for example, will suck out a 'ransong', a type of object that has been placed in the body by a hostile source and that causes intense pain.[5] When we start to think more generally of the new genetics as an ethno-ethics of divination in lieu of the more familiar understanding of genetic science as decoding work, we can see that biological 'interiority' as a hidden dimension of reality does not necessarily occlude other kinds of *social anatomies* (see Chapter 2). But the comparisons cannot be left there. Atkinson (1989:118) remarks that although health and life depend on the concentration of vital elements of being, there appears to be nothing that holds a person together from within. Clearly there is a difference between this indigenous vision of personhood and the cultural imaginary by which Westerners commonly imagine themselves as internally bound through the integral properties of spiralling matter – the folk wisdom of the biochemical constituents of DNA code. But are things really so very different between these respective visions of bodily constitution? Atkinson's conclusive point is that Wana health and sociality turn out to be intricately linked insofar as one's general well being will always depend on an ethic of interdependence. This is the point she explores throughout her analysis of Wana personhood whose creative expression is given voice through 'an anatomy of dependence'. 'Rather than managing these [corporeal] elements on one's own, a person must submit to the care of a specialist who can know more about one's ultimate state of being than one can know oneself. In this way, dependence on shamanic mediation *is built into the very constitution of the person*' (Atkinson 1989:119, emphasis added). By citing the extended pre-symptomatic illness narratives and moral trajectories of several Hungtington's families, the point is not how British kin engage spirit familiars even if we can see why predictive genetic testing technology invites interesting parallels with the oracular gaze of divinatory power. It is rather how the value of genetic information that now relates so much more explicitly to Westerners conceptions of 'self' is something that may be recognised as the activation of social anatomies of interdependence.

Drawing upon case studies of the two families, we have seen how shifting affiliations between kin do not *necessarily* divide neatly along lines of shared genetic inheritance. Identifying the phenomena of 'siding' as one significant strategy for dealing with new genetic knowledge, there are a number of points to observe about these emergent forms of kinship as processes of pre-symptomatic value reckoning. First, though 'siding' with like-tested kin involves implicit alliances that may have nothing necessarily to do with notions of 'blood' (consanguineal) relatedness, family relations may take the form of reproducing others as 'excluded' relatedness. Kin may become 'outsiders within' as we saw in the first example (Kingston/Richardson family); a situation that was resolved through a family dispute in the second example (Williams family). Second, idealistic notions of the family as 'safe haven' underscore much of the 'non-directive' counselling of health professionals. Without probing how pre-symptomatic persons form part of a complex network of interdependent relations and thus comprise a vital cosmology of 'social anatomy', genetic counsellors and others in the policy field risk perpetuating misplaced stereotypes of 'the family' as homogenous self-referential unit (see Chapter 4). People may well resist the way others have transformed them into morally engaged 'prophylactic agents', but conflicts of interest between kin may be evident not only as divergence (forms of exclusion selection); they may also be about settling kinship equivalence as parities of doubt. Such practice fundamentally challenges (1) the sociobiological doctrine of 'inclusive fitness' and the kin selection thesis of genetic fetishism and gene replicability; and (2) the neo-liberal premise of the value of personhood as individual autonomy that underpins mainstream bioethics conceptualisations of the right to know/right not to know debates. Framed within a cross-cultural or ethno-ethical perspective, the 'inventiveness' of Western genetics' own theoretical corpus starts to look less fabulous against a wealth of local detail informing other folk theories of the origins of life. It also looks decidedly pale when held up against non-Western indigenous practices of divination that point to the shaman or healer's expertise concerning sources of misfortune and affliction, as well as to the way that these practices reflect local theories about relationships between people and the wider social community. As we shall see in the next chapter, the negotiation of competing interests between kin is yet more explicit as forms of cultural 'selection' in the area of genetics and reproductive decision-making.

6

Relinquishing exclusion

Let me begin with a little cautionary tale about exclusion testing. As a story within a story, there is a Russian Doll effect. But all is not what it seems. Orientation: we will be circling first of all around a sub-text whose plot prises open the problem of the 'mock embryo transfer'.

Pre-implanting a story

Novel preconception testing technology such as pre-implantation genetic diagnosis (PGD) offers – the interested patient is told – a treatment procedure for those couples who want to have children without the potential risk of transmitting a pre-diagnosed hereditary condition to their offspring.[1] Parents-to-be who may be considering such 'treatment' will be informed further by clinicians that the technique allows them to start a pregnancy with a pre-selected healthy embryo. Prospective PGD patients will be given statistics and risk figures that put the option of pre-implantation diagnosis into context, as against leaving things to nature and having a non-assisted conception. The medical assumption that a single cell diagnosis is ethically preferable to the elective termination of a pregnancy after prenatal diagnosis (or spontaneous termination) – something this group of patients is also likely to be told (or may know intuitively) – is an explanatory narrative that legitimises novel methods of human conception. It is therefore a moral narrative of a kind, framed as it is around certain 'quality of life' beliefs and sensibilities. For those committed clinicians specialising in the field of PGD services, a strong sense of professional satisfaction is derived from their ability to assist couples in their quest to reproduce healthy children. But these clinicians' narratives – the words that accompany their clinical skill and acts of professional judgement – are usually less explicit in their moral accounting of the possible unintended consequences these interventions effect beyond

124

the treatment regimen of any one given couple. For just as parents can be seen to reproduce offspring in new ways, so novel preconception testing technologies such as pre-implantation genetic diagnosis can be said to reproduce 'society' in unexpected ways.

An embryo that has been 'selected out' as potentially viable for future life in comparison with others that have been screened and put aside, donated to research or discarded. This is what the genetic diagnosis of a potential person (as the 'pre-embryo' entity) at the pre-implantation stage entails. PGD techniques combine developments in new reproductive and genetic screening technologies, specifically *in-vitro* fertilisation (IVF) and genetically determined selection or prioritisation, in order to make prospective life and death decisions about human viability. Crucially, these genetic decisions are made before a woman conceives and starts the maternal work of gestation. Contrary to prenatal diagnosis technologies, the prospective parents face the 'choice' of beginning a pregnancy with the foreknowledge that only genetically unaffected embryos will have the chance of surviving as potential life form. PGD testing technology thus enables the creation of a certain iconographic time-space within clinical worlds. In the abstract, the extra-corporeal exclusion of the pre-conceived embryo as a viable kinship entity for future relationality can be rationalised (by professionals and others) as though the act of selecting-out is a 'natural' part of the human 'assisted' (IVF) reproductive process. 'Choice' in other words becomes fetishised and routinised; it is gradually encultured as a normal part of the process to parenthood, just like the technologies themselves that are said to facilitate such 'normalised' selection processes (cf. Browner and Press 1995; Press and Browner 1994 on the routinisation of prenatal testing technologies). But this capacity for procreative agents (potential parents and health practitioners) to intervene culturally in the time prior to the maternal implantation of the embryo renders genetic decision-making particularly fraught. The PGD iconography has other embodied versions too.

In the case of anticipating the presence of a late-onset symptomatology such as Huntington's Disease, predictive pre-implantation genetic testing turns on having to decide whether it can ever be justifiable to end a potential life that would not actually be seen to manifest symptoms for several decades after birth. In biomedical terms, and also in moral philosophical terms, such decisions are seen to require principles, norms and pre-defined guidelines for action. It is not uncommon for particularly intransigent ethical dilemmas such as these also to provoke the generation of euphemisms. Deciding whether it can ever be justifiable to end a potential life may transmute into an eventuality that is elided discursively in the biomedical realm with the terms 'exclusion PGD testing' or 'prenatal exclusion test' for example (see Braude *et al.* 1998; Tyler *et al.* 1990).

Through the technical provision of pre-emptive 'exclusion' as a morally valid procedure and categorisation, PGD technology presumes then the evaluation of a prior judgement. It presumes that we as a society have evaluated already more than just what it means to be genetically constituted as a pre-symptomatic human being. It demands of us that we are able to discriminate what kinds of moralities can go towards making up the very idea of the 'pre-symptomatic' person as a specific cultural imaginary.

But pre-implantation testing techniques not only discriminate pre-conceptively between so-called viable and non-viable forms of human life, they may also evoke an elaborate constellation of *secret* claims to knowledge within the moral space of the clinic. As discretionary knowledge flows, such genetic information is converted into intricately nested forms of concealment whose moral power resides in the fact that forms of non-knowledge circulate between numerous health professionals, the prospective parents and the 'elusive' entity of the (pre) embryo.[2] So-called 'non-disclosure PGD' (Schulmann *et al.* 1996; Braude *et al.* 1998; cf. Sermon *et al.* 1998) aims to protect informational privacy by inhibiting the evident implication of biologically related kin in others' genetic information. For those prospective parents who know they are 'at risk' but crucially who do not want to have their own genetic status made *less* ambivalent (i.e. verified as positive or negative) through the selective screening procedures, pre-implantation diagnosis by non-disclosure effectively cuts off the flow of genetic information. During counselling sessions such pre-consenting couples are told that it will be 'safe' for them to undergo IVF with pre-implantation embryo biopsy/testing as specific genetic test results will be withheld from them, thus making it impossible to access any potentially revealing information about themselves and their heredity. Throughout the procedure, and afterwards, neither of the two biological parents are able to receive any information about the number of oocytes that have been obtained from the mother-to-be after hormonal stimulation and 'pick-up' retrieval. Nor are any details made available about the number of embryos that have been tested and deemed suitable for procreative transfer to the mother.

But 'non-disclosure PGD testing', as a clinical variation of 'exclusion PGD testing' and 'prenatal exclusion testing'[3] is seen to raise many ethical concerns. In particular, a number of health professionals have questioned the extent to which non-disclosure may violate the bioethical principle of non-maleficence. This refers to the medical obligation to avoid inflicting harm on the patient(s) – in these cases, namely the mother and her IVF-cultured embryo(s). For our purposes, one of the main problems concerns non-disclosure as an embodied and interrelational practice of 'social anatomy' (see Chapter 5). At various points in the treatment, it is in fact possible for patients to infer from the success or otherwise of their PGD cycles whether or not they are a-symptomatic 'carriers'.

On many counts, eliminating exclusion by implication turns out to be a morally delicate as well as procedurally tricky technique to perform. As one treatment team explains, when there are no unaffected embryos to transfer 'the doctors could feel compelled to conduct *a mock embryo transfer* in order to maintain the deception required for non-disclosure' (Braude *et al.* 1998:1424–25, emphasis added). Writing in their capacity as practising clinicians, the authors go on to explain various permutations of the deceptive 'pretence'. If the expected transfer procedure fails to materialise, a potential parent may assume rightly or wrongly that they carry the mutation in question, even if they have received genetic counselling to the contrary. Since there can be genuinely plausible non-genetic reasons why no 'healthy' embryos manage to survive for corporeal transfer – due to failure of embryonic fertilisation or cleavage, for example – it may well be the case that the parents end up worrying about a non-conception for no good cause. For those couples who do not conceive successfully after embryo transfer, yet in fact have generated non 'carrier' (i.e. unaffected) embryos, 'the pretence' would nonetheless have to be maintained since 'tell[ing] the client this 'good news' would constitute a breach of non-disclosure' (*ibid*, p. 1425) Furthermore, hypothetical disclosure to non-affected parents 'would also be an indirect and unintended breach of *other* at-risk clients' right not to know' (Braude *et al.* 1998:1426; emphasis added). With this last point the PGD experts effectively confirm the view that heredity, as an immanent ethics of kinship disclosure, cannot be conceived simply as the objectified abstractions of a single person or family's medical genealogy. Prospective parents with 'good' news forfeit the knowledge they are not pre-symptomatic and are positioned as coeval with other presenting (and non-identifiable) parents similarly protective of the preferred entitlement 'not to know'. Now these parents may be strangers to one another but through these techniques they are brought together as linked testing candidates whose futures become intertwined. These parents' reproductive choices are social anatomies: they actively make relations of interdependence. In the decision-making space of the genetics clinic, these moral interests will be run together as simultaneous versions of the same social complex: the prevarication over how much genetic knowledge it is imagined it is good to know and from what source.

Note however that there are usually considerable logistical difficulties for maintaining secrecy within a PGD multidisciplinary treatment team (see Sermon *et al.* 1998; Braude *et al.* 1998). The doctor, the embryologist, the nurses and anaesthetist may all know the number of oocytes that have been collected from a given woman's uterus as each follicle is drained and placed in culture. Almost certainly the principal embryologist will know the fertilisation rate and how many embryos were suitable for cell biopsy and testing in each patient's case. Also, it is not unusual for a number of different consultants to be engaged with the oocyte retrieval stage and embryo transfer part of the process. In other words, members of a clinical team are more rather than less likely to find out sooner or later the adult patient's carrier status. The problem of unintentional disclosure and information leaks thus sets up a moral genealogy and exchange form of its own: the career life of the secret that travels within the confines of the professional clinic setting. An important consideration is whether patients known by at least one member of the multidisciplinary team *not* to be an affected carrier can be 'supported' through such physically, emotionally and financially demanding treatment procedures (Sermon *et al.* 1998).[4] As already mentioned, for those people who turn out not to carry the defective gene, PGD treatment (involving IVF hormonal stimulation through high doses of drugs and other attendant risks) turns out to be a treatment that is completely unnecessary. And yet the conundrum of this reproductive 'net' is difficult to renege: it generates its own relations of interdependence since for staff to refuse a determined couple a further course of IVF treatment sometime in the future would constitute in itself an act of unintended disclosure.[5] Keeping up the 'pretence' (Braude *et al.* 1998:1425) so that people will not be able to infer their 'at risk' status from what does not happen is a deception that turns the technical procedure of PGD into something of a piece with a 'treatment fiction'.

From another viewpoint, these practices of non-disclosure unwittingly implicate the pre-symptomatic figure of the pre-embryo in the mediations of an 'open secret' (cf. Chapter 4) between the various laboratory technicians and other medical staff. Situated between life and death, the pre-conceived pre-embryo elusively 'reproduces' for its parents-to-be the continued prerogative not to know what could be unwanted genetic information about a past maternal or paternal inheritance. Through the exclusions offered by the clinic, set up and operationalised as its expert technical knowledge, prospective parents and prospective child are grown and grow each other within the informational folds of a mutually secretive skein of knowledge and non-knowledge (see discussion of McCallum's work in Chapter 4). It is from out of these entangled folds that each stands to the other as procreative and interdependent co-partner(s).[6] If the embryo is tested and found positive, then the parental decision not to perform a termination transforms the potential child into a person who has been born 'pre-symptomatic' without his or her prior consent to the social facilitation of such knowledge. Mainstream bioethicists and others are wont to deflect such interdependence as violations of a person's individual autonomy. Potentiation, however, refers not just to what contract theorists and others will see as missed conceptions, misconceptions or even 'contested' conceptions. Each relation (mother/pre-embryo and pre-embryo/mother) projects the other as its responsible agency: the parents stand to reproduce the foetus as the foetus 'reproduces' (its) parents: a classic holographic inversion that sees interdependent persons as 'nested' relations.[7] In juxtaposing here some excerpts from women's own highly intimate reproductive and parenting testimonies, the following two vignettes probe further why and how these exclusionary technologies might sometimes meet public resistance through acts of maternal refusal.

"Treading together ... I'd rather them all be in the same boat"

Since Daisy already knew she was HD positive when she was expecting her daughters Rosa and Penny, PGD exclusion testing by non-disclosure was not a viable alternative for her as no information would have been lost. Prior to the birth of her eldest child, Jamie, preconceptive exclusion testing had not been medically available and thus was not a reproductive option. However, before she fell pregnant for the first time, Daisy could have decided to go for a direct predictive test herself since the family secret about her mother's diagnosed HD had been disclosed some time previously (see Chapter 4). With the second so-called 'accidental' pregnancy (Rosa's birth), prenatal exclusion testing of the foetus was still an option for her had she so wished, and with her last pregnancy (Penny), she could have chosen between pre-implantation genetic diagnosis and prenatal exclusion testing. By juxtaposing these various procreative options as the past subjunctives of genetically informed 'choices', it is possible to see how Daisy's decision-making sets up an affective trail of kinship reckoning as a local instantiation of a genealogical ethics. In the following section of dialogue, excerpted from a longer conversation, Daisy articulates why a selective abortion or other pre-conceptive 'terminations' would not necessarily lighten her family's load should any of her children turn out to be HD-affected in the future. She begins by explaining she was pregnant with Rosa at the time she received her positive test result.

MK: So at the time that you had the predictive test you were already pregnant. Was that it?

DO: Yeah, we'd sort of found out at the same sort of time. She was an accident (giggling). We found out at the time of the tests that I was expecting.

MK: So what did the genetic counsellor say to you about that, that you were coming for the test and expecting Rosa?

DO: They didn't know until I had the test result. I think we found out a couple of days before we had the positive test back. I didn't actually say anything. My first feelings were "Do we have this baby? Do we have the foetal test? Do we abort? Or, you know, do we carry on sort of thing?" It was a real muddle.

MK: What was that like? Finding out that you were pregnant just a few days before you had your own test result back?

DO: Terrible. It was almost like "Oh my God, what have I done to these children?" You know. "I can't believe I've done this. I've done it to Jamie. I don't want to do it to another child". That was my first reaction. "I could have destroyed your life, I suppose" but . . . I went away and spoke to my sister and she said, "Well at the end of the day do you regret the life you've had?" and I said, "Well, no" and she said, "Would you rather have not been born?" And I said "No" and she said, "Well, there you go then" and I thought, "Well, yes you're right", you know.

MK: When you got the results in the clinic did you tell them there that you just had a pregnancy test confirmed?

DO: No.

MK: Do you remember how you felt? What thoughts were going through your mind when you got the result then about your positive test and what this would mean later . . . having Huntington's?

DO: "My God, what are we going to do?", I think [chuckles]

MK: Yes. Was there, was there any particular reason why you didn't want to go ahead with the baby?

DO: I suppose because in the back of my mind I was thinking "Should we go ahead with it?". And if I had a termination I wouldn't, you know, I wouldn't want to have done it then or go back and sort of later . . . I don't know, I just needed time for it all to sink in and become real. And I think in early pregnancy it hadn't sunk in at all about my baby. Even later stages of pregnancy it's like, you know, four or five months later it hadn't . . . . It's almost not real at all. It's really hard to come to sort of terms with the pregnancy, let alone knowing you've got something like that happening.

MK: So then did you think about the questions that they probably would have put to you if you had told them at the clinic you were expecting?

DO: I was worried that they were going to think I was wrong for having the children.

MK: That they'd be judgmental, that sort of thing?

DO: Yeah, yeah I thought they would be. You know, because like my first contact with a doctor was at a GP and he wasn't my own GP. And when I first mentioned it to him that I found out about this [the HD] and what shall I do? His first reaction was like "Oh well it's hereditary. They'll probably advise you not to have children". And it was just like it was all so clear-cut. And he sat there with his children's pictures on his desk.

This was before I'd had any [children]. I'd lost a baby, the first baby that I was carrying. And it was just like so cold that I come out of there and I was a complete wreck. This was before I had got the test result [for HD]. All I ever wanted was to be a mum and that was it. Gone, you know. I didn't want anybody to tell me "No you can't do this".

MK: Yes.

DO: And then, you know, I knew that the people-testing thing was being started. But then there's also the risk of miscarriage. And I said to Greg "What if we had the test and it was negative" you know what I mean? And then you miscarry. It would be like a double disaster. You know? We'd be losing a healthy child.

MK: Yes, I . . .

DO: And then I thought "Oh, we've got one child at risk". How can I say to him later in life: "I'm sorry Jamie, but you're at risk and your siblings aren't". I'd rather them all be in the same boat and all be there to protect each other rather than having one all by himself with this thing, you know. . . . I don't think it was fair to stop the others getting it if I couldn't do that for Jamie, I suppose.

MK: How do you mean?

DO: Well, he was the only one not definitely negative. And I thought how can I take him away from his siblings and say, "Well you're the only one that's at risk". Rather than sitting them all down and saying "Well look this is and . . .". It just didn't seem fair on him at all, you know.

MK: Yes. So were you really thinking then at this stage about Rosa in terms of the future relations between the two siblings?

DO: Yes yeah. It's almost like now they're all in the same boat. They've all been treated exactly the same. So they can all support each other because they're all going to be feeling the same feelings. They're all in the same situation. Whereas if I'd had the other two tested and I knew they were both negative and I had this one child with a question mark, it wouldn't have been right.

MK: So you wanted some kind of equivalence between . . .

DO: Yes. It's almost like with our family, you know. Me and me sister, Liz, it's almost like we've got this thing and I . . . it's pulling us together. We're supporting each other through it. Whereas I think if it was just me and I knew Liz was negative, I would almost back away from her, rather then pull together. I'd be like "Well you don't understand. Just leave me alone". Whereas she does understand.

MK: Even though if she does have a test later on it might be different from yours?

DO: Yeah, well I'm sure she probably is okay actually. The nurse was saying she's not showing any obvious signs, you know. I'm sure she probably is [okay]. But it's the fact that we've been in the same boat and she's got that worry. Whereas if she was negative she wouldn't understand how I was feeling at all. And she's convinced she's positive. She's feeling exactly the same things as I am so we're treading together.

Daisy thinks that if only one of her children were known to be at risk of having inherited a genetic predisposition for an illness with delayed symptomatology, it would be unfair to exclude the probability of that same risk applying to subsequent offspring too. It would not be fair 'to stop the others getting it if I couldn't do that for Jamie', she says. He is the '. . . only one not definitely negative . . . how can I take him away from the rest of the siblings? This notion of sibling equivalence as kin inclusiveness projected forward onto future relationality between as yet unborn and existing child(ren) is modelled on the selective avoidance of these advanced PGD preconception technologies. This sensibility of 'evening-up' the distribution of genetic risk between siblings came up again with other parents and siblings, though I would want to stress that such views are not the understandings of all couples. Indeed I am not in a position to evaluate the representative status of the stories I tell, only to know that these may be unusual though by no means exceptional cases.[8] Certainly a sense of anticipating the social meaning of genetic ties in this way builds in additional kinship factors about what it means to create a new taxonomy of 'pre-symptomatic' persons as differentiated degrees of relatedness. The narratives speak therefore to what are perhaps incipient ideas of kin inclusiveness in these new familial contexts. They tell us about the desirability of relinquishing exclusion and the social inequity of testing cultures, as this is perceived by some who are directly affected by these innovative predictive technologies. But what exactly are these beliefs? Some parents who consider it unacceptable to 'mix' siblings according to the different genetic status of their children's future susceptibility to risk are saying that the intentional procreation of differently constituted siblings would endow one child with fixed privilege. It would be like the 'pre-conception' of a socially favoured sibling – if not necessarily in their own eyes, then in terms of how parents anticipate others will look upon the family as 'outsiders' and discern them in the literal sense of being 'set apart' – seen with discrimination.[9] It is hard to know whether these are retrospective justifications put forward 'after the event' of birth to appease Daisy's feelings of guilt, or whether such reasoning actively shaped her pre-conceptive decision-making each time she conceived. In any case, through her refusal to take up the clinical offers of prenatal monitoring and intervention, she effectively 'stills' the technology of embryonic selection and selective abortion. In her own way she terminates or 'finishes off' the choice of 'exclusion' as a meaningful procreative possibility for her family. These attempts to 'still' choice can also be seen as ways of activating heredity as techniques of 'de-selection'. Such 'de-selection' techniques can be compared with other recent ethnographic evidence documenting the active strategies of pregnant women and their partners to refuse prenatal diagnosis in other prophylactic and genetic surveillance contexts (see Rapp 2000; Asch 1999; cf. Beeson and Doksum's [2001] analysis of 'experiential resistance'). A connection can also be made with the voices of certain disability lobbyists campaigning for the right to ensure their children may be born with the *same* inherited disability as themselves. In the UK, for example, the 'right' of parents to choose preferentially those embryos affected by their own genetic disorder has been considered tentatively in the case of so-called 'mild' disability.[10]

In contexts such as these, the ideal of sibling equivalence may also be preferred because it is seen to excuse the pre-symptomatic parent's perceived obligation to have to tell children they are 'at risk'. Daisy upholds the imagined possibilities of kin inclusiveness because she does not want to be morally complicit in having co-created genetic foreknowledge about her children *on their behalf*. This is a 'choice' that unfolds around an appreciation of tentative genealogy as degrees of relative uncertainty. It is better, she thinks, that the siblings remain 'risk-related' than that she should pre-empt their misfortune by having herself directly tested first. Parent and offspring, in this sense, are 'nested' universes each containing within itself a miniature constellation of the other as a series of generative possibilities. Crucially, these generative possibilities enjoin particular genealogical discernments. Referring back to our conversation, which in real-time follows on some time later on from the previous excerpted dialogue, comparisons with the techniques of prenatal diagnosis are introduced by me into the discussion.

MK: Would you have wanted to have a prenatal test for HD if they had said to you that it's up to you if you have a test to find out whether the foetus is affected, but there's absolutely no pressure to have a selective termination.

DO: No.

MK: That you can know if you'd wanted to?

DO: No because that spells looking into other people's life. It's got to be their choice when they're older of whether they want to know. I couldn't live my life with them wondering about it and me knowing.

MK: How do you mean?

DO: Well if the baby's positive, then I'd carried on and given birth to that baby.

MK: I see, yes.

DO: I couldn't live every day looking at the child knowing that I know the secret. It wouldn't be right. It would almost be like this thing of not telling the truth. And having them going through, you know, the teenage years and wondering about it. I couldn't sit there, and pretend I didn't know. And that to me isn't . . . I'm not the person that should be telling them. You know, they need to find out for themselves when and if they want to. At the time that suits them, not the time that suits me.

Daisy's narration of genealogical reckoning highlights that other reproductive trajectories *could have* shaped the mother-foetus/foetus-mother's self-actualisation and how such subjunctive trajectories are transformed by her into meaningful knowledge that is both lost or 'de-conceived' as well as open to subsequent retrieval. (Namely, knowledge can be re-conceived later by others as a relational claim of intergenerational justice, or wrongful life for example.) This is an altogether different form of 'active forgetting' to that propagated by the clinic (see above 'pre-implanting a story'). There, concealment was traced by stealth and the secret of the transfer of the 'mock embryo' became part of the career trajectories of institutionalised exclusions that justify a scientific 'anatomy of ignorance' as disembodied non-disclosure. Daisy doesn't want to carry the awful burden of knowledge that comes with 'looking into other people's life'. Hers is an active embodied refusal of genetic knowledge that delimits parental obligation by scoping the nature of maternal responsibility through understandings of kin inclusiveness. The lesson of her story? The idea of belonging to a particular family that defines itself, at least in part, through its shared experience of collective illness susceptibility, that copes with adversity and gets by, is a more appealing version of the 'truth' to inhabit, than deceptive pretences that eradicate the context of life and living altogether.

De-selecting life and redescribing relative disloyalties

Sibling equivalence and obligations to existing offspring

When Isobel is told about the news contained in Oliver's letter (see Chapter 4), she happens herself to have found out only a few days beforehand that she is six weeks pregnant. As it happens, Bruno's parents, her in-laws, have not had this news disclosed to them before they decide to make known their own distressing announcement.[11] Isobel had felt anger and frustration upon finding herself pregnant with Louise at just the time Bruno's health became a matter of serious family concern and medical investigation. Not having gone ahead with prenatal testing for Stefan is something she has since regretted, and as she explains: '. . . [it is] not because I would have gone for termination had the foetus been affected . . . but *I think I just would have preferred to have known then*' (emphasis added). Stressing that she would not have wanted to go ahead with prenatal testing for the sake of excluding an embryo whose genetic make-up revealed the presence of Down's or HD, she explains that now from a retrospective vantage it would have been preferable to take up the offer of screening. She wishes she had gone ahead with the tests simply so as to know (already at that time) whether or not her second child may develop HD. As we shall see, Isobel – contrary to Daisy – finds the frustration of now not knowing certain genetic details about her children an impractical, painfully intolerable and inflexible prohibition.

ID: I mean we were talking about having tests with Louisa for probably two months. Because at that time they could test whether the child was tentative [?] within the womb. If I would have had the test, I would know today whether she was carrying Huntington's. But now it's got to be the professionals' opinion.

MK: Would you mind just going through that so that I can get what the difference was?

ID: If we took having had Stefan, then having another Down's child wouldn't have been a problem. Stefan is Stefan and to have an abortion or whatever just because the child was disabled, no. Maybe it was like a guilt thing, if you had one child then you got rid of another. You would not be fair to the child.

MK: Which child?

ID: Stefan. If we had the testing done. Because it shouldn't be. But hospitals assume if you have the test done, then you are going to abort if it is not right. And I had the blood test done and they were very reluctant to do them. I wanted to know the risk, to prepare, because of the reactions we had had from the family when Stefan was born. To prepare them again. You could see the look on their faces . . . "We can only give you a percentage", they were saying. The look on their faces, of that kind of horror, you know, when I said I would keep . . . nothing aborted.

MK: You were saying that Down's wasn't the issue?

ID: The child being disabled wasn't the issue. The difference I suppose, it's also what my conscience was saying to me. It is almost as if you had an abortion for one child, and you . . . I know that child was never likely to grow up understanding what you have done, but it's as if you don't really want that child there if you had been given a choice.

MK: How so, do you mean?

ID: It is almost like a disloyalty to Stefan. It's as if we say, "Well, we really didn't want you, you were a problem really". But it wouldn't be. I did not do it thinking, "That cannot happen to us again". I was well aware that it could happen. That you could end up with two children, I mean it really didn't need to be bad, it could have been another issue. But to this day I do regret not taking the test. It was offered and again it was a conscious . . . it would have been a risk to the baby, and I didn't really think what this could hold for the future.

MK: So were you wanting to have the test for the HD?

ID: At the time, no. Because I didn't understand the consequences of not having it done. I mean I don't know what I would have done if it had been positive. If it meant . . . having an abortion. I would look at the children and I live in hope that there is going to be something to help them before they developed it. And I am just praying that they are not the unlucky children that develop it in childhood. And the professionals say to me "Well, the children probably won't develop it". But the more I go into things, the more I am becoming aware that children do develop it and there are more children today with it. I know what they are saying, and you know I have even said to them I want . . . I don't know, but I am so frustrated at the fact that if we had have had that test we would have sat here knowing today whether Louisa carried the gene or didn't carry the gene.

The orthodox biomedical view assumes that if a couple already have an affected child, or have had one or more terminations because of a genetic disorder in the foetus, they may feel less able to cope with the demands of another affected child, or a further termination (Human Fertilisation and Embryology Authority/Advisory Committee on Genetic Testing 1999:9).[12] These assumptions, in turn, are premised on the biomedical calculation of risk as statistical measurements of probability and on conceptions of the person as singular, self-bounded and autonomous. Isobel explained to me that the clinical team in charge of her care was reluctant to carry out prenatal screening since she had already indicated that she would not want to terminate irrespective of the test result findings. Such reports reinforce other women's accounts of the subtle and sometimes less subtle pressures exerted on them by medics to agree beforehand not to continue with their pregnancy should their foetus show up a genetic impairment. Termination, though, can be presented as a 'sanitised' act, you can be told or guided or directed that it is what others in your situation would reasonably do. Alternatively, the agony of decision-making some parents go through over whether or not to terminate can be countered by the 'benefits' of pre-implantation diagnosis: in-built into the PGD procedure itself are prior substitutions and the knowledge that parents have (had) that decision removed for them. As one senior genetic counsellor working at a large genetics unit explained to Huntington's couples: 'Until recently an individual who is at risk of, or has Huntington's disease and wishes to have a baby who will not inherit the condition, could opt to have a test during their pregnancy. This form of testing is called prenatal diagnosis. If a pregnancy was found to have inherited the gene, then the couple would usually opt to terminate the pregnancy'.[13] In practice however parental decision-making may be compounded by additional anxieties over the nature of parental responsibility in the light of newly available genetic knowledge afforded by these technologies. Commenting on the protocol for prenatal tests and pre-implantation diagnosis, a government consultation paper on genetic testing and late-onset illness states: 'A particular issue arises when a couple decide to continue a pregnancy after an abnormal prenatal test result. This effectively gives pre-symptomatic diagnosis for the child after it is born . . .' (ACGT 1997:24). With this statement we can see the presumption of at least two key objections: first, for a woman to resist termination threatens to undermine the whole rationale of prenatal screening itself. Why do the testing if you are not going to screen out the deformity you find? (Indeed these are precisely Isobel's worst fears.) And second, there is the presumption of the violation of the principle of informed consent. The premise here is that the birth of an affected child after genetic testing transforms the foetus into a cultural entity that did not give personal consent to this knowledge being created for and about itself. Here parents can be seen to implicate themselves morally as social agents of 'unsolicited disclosure', as discussed at length in Chapter 4. A pregnant woman who decides against abortion, and in cases where no treatment intervention is available, should also be aware that 'any child born will not have the option of deciding not to be tested' (Nuffield Council on Bioethics 1998:47).[14]

Evidence, however, from a recent opinion poll in the UK on public attitudes to genetic information reveals that more respondents tended to disagree with the statement that persons 'at risk of having a child with a serious genetic disorder' should be discouraged from having children of their own (HGC 2001:58). For

Isobel's part, not testing Louisa prenatally for HD is transposed into an act of maternal 'loyalty' to Stefan, the couple's eldest 'at risk' child. Were a pregnancy to be excluded preferentially, it is as though the parent retrospectively transmits unequal kinship emotion to existing offspring: it is tantamount to saying that already the child-to-be could also have been aborted as a worthless life. Such maternal acts of inclusiveness have the effect of 'stilling' technologies of selection. Expressed as sentiments of kin loyalty, de-selecting life 'aborts' exclusion testing as legitimate technique.[15] Another way of saying this is to see the practice of 'relinquishing exclusion' as one constitutive act of a relational ethics. Through refusal, one actively makes social anatomies of interdependence. These anatomies may be durable, fractious and weak, but they are always social; they elicit relationality within or across the generations. In the particular examples discussed here, offspring are not simply pre-conceived by parents and others as physical representations of the biological engendering of life. Children, rather, are actively *pre-imagined* as certain kinship relations. Offspring-to-be are implicated as kin since they evolve from an anticipatory form of equivalence whereby their 'separateness' as human persons is already prospectively embodied as interrelationship prior to the actual physiological event of birth itself. As Rayna Rapp (1999:189) observes in the context of North American women's experiences of amniocentesis: 'Those who opt to continue a pregnancy after any positive diagnosis must consciously face what the rest of us confront only episodically: The hard work of redescribing and reinscribing a powerful biomedical definition into the more complex and variegated aspects of personhood, childhood dependency, and family life'. While the ideal of sibling equivalence may be one motivational factor for 'stilling' selection within genetically risk susceptible families, there may be contexts when parents and others feel a need to justify what they perceive as meaningful differences between potentially pre-symptomatic kin. There are not simply 'gaps', as Rapp (1999:175–78) rightly describes, between biomedical diagnoses and the integration of diagnosed babies into family life; there are subtle shifts of allegiance and social anatomy formation *within* families. I found Isobel one interlocutor prepared to be refreshingly honest with her 'confessions' of maternal favouritism. Her articulations, though, are likely to expose her to moral opprobrium from critics who would see her stratified attentions and description of care-giving as evidence of 'bad' mothering. Her narrative is thus acutely vulnerable to possible misinterpretation by the biomedical complex and others who would castigate what they see as a morally 'dangerous' lack of maternal love. Remember too that Isobel represents the relatively privileged voice of the white, middle-class, well-educated woman. Others may stand to be misinterpreted far more readily.

"I treat my children differently anyway"

Since the birth of her second child and Bruno's diagnosis, Isobel has taken on board more fully the implications of living her future within a pre-symptomatic household and thinks it in the best interests of her family for the children to be tested before they reach their eighteenth birthdays. As just mentioned, she originally had refused prenatal genetic testing for Louisa because, so far as she was concerned, there was never any question of Isobel undergoing a termination. This is not to say that foreknowledge of the illness would not have been 'helpful' information, she further explains – at least in terms of her being able to make practical plans about future care arrangements and other eventualities.

Mainstream professional opinion amongst clinical geneticists in the UK has cautioned against the testing of children for adult onset conditions, mainly on the grounds that the information to be gained would not have any benefit for the individual during childhood years.[16] Almost uniformly, the interpretive framing device has been guided by appeal to the notion of the 'best interests' of the child. There is also the related objection that testing before the age of eighteen denies the child the chance of making their own autonomous choice as an adult – precisely the problem that non-termination after prenatal exclusion testing sets up. Health policy makers, genetic counsellors and others in the child welfare field have also expressed considerable concern that such information, once revealed, could lead to forms of discrimination in the family. Having requested 'juvenile genetic testing' Isobel has encountered strong medical resistance to the idea and talks indignantly about the medics' reprisal that testing would make her children 'different' from their peers. In the following excerpt, I'm asking her a speculative question about another form of difference: genetic information as knowledge unevenly distributed between her two children. At this point in our conversation I was interested to find out her views should only one child have been tested – Louisa, her second born. How, I wondered, did she imagine this as a series of kin obligations and moral exigencies? Our discussion leads to some reflections on forms of familial 'discrimination'.

MK: What would that knowledge have set up in terms of knowing about one of the children but not the other? Not knowing about Stefan?

ID: Then I would have pushed harder to have Stefan[tested], because there was a big query over him and I am still pushing. Sometimes I wonder why I am doing it because what good would it do? I have been trying for a long time but it is not legally [possible]. It's financially going through more. We couldn't afford to do it [privately]. And the time before they can see in the future that it is probably going to be necessary, because my argument is when he reaches eighteen, my rights as parent even though

he is disabled are going to be taken away, and that decision will never
be made.

MK: Which decision?

ID: Because . . . I am playing God here. I have some idea as to what ability
Stefan has, just looking at him and seeing how he is going along. When
he is eighteen he is not going to be able to . . . He may understand that
Daddy is disabled, if he [Bruno] is still alive. He may understand that he
is disabled, but to sit him down with facts on Huntington's. I'm afraid
his disability . . . and knowing that he can still learn but he is not going
to learn to the degree that maybe Louisa will learn, the understanding
of it. And I can see . . . I am always going to have to be aware of
where Stefan is and what he is doing, and we are looking for community
care of some sort for him in the future. But if he was going to have to
have a member of the family or a trustee to take care of his personal
finances, or whatever, and I hope that he is going to have some nephews
or nieces to keep an eye on him. Not take care of him. Just make sure
that he is being treated properly. Where he goes, what he does, and how
he is treated are . . . if he is carrying the gene for Huntington's, or if he
is going to develop it, I feel they have the right to know. I mean, the
[medical] argument is that people will treat him differently. I treat my
children differently anyway . . . I am a lot harder on him because he has
to be . . . society is hard on him anyway. If we are out in public, and
starts doing things he shouldn't do, then society assumes he is not being
childlike, he is doing that because he is 'Down's'. I just . . . [breaking
down, crying] . . . I just feel that people are going to be looking after, I
mean, I could go tomorrow and somebody is going to have to take care
of him. I mean our grandparents won't be able to. So my argument is I
should be allowed to prepare, to put into writing, what I want for him.

When he comes to eighteen, though he is disabled, he becomes an
adult in his own right, and nobody is going to hand that responsibility
over to the social workers, to the professionals. And I feel that is not
what I want. I just care deeply to what is going to happen to them and
yes, I know we cannot do anything . . . It's information, you know, I just
feel the need for a . . . to have that information . . . society does treat
him differently anyway. They shouldn't do, but they do. Whether it is
the fact that he is going to develop HD. And again, that's my argument
talking to Professor B. and the team at the clinic.

MK: So what ideally would you like? For Stefan to be tested first?

ID: I would like for them both to be done, I mean yes, I feel that I would
need counselling and Bruno would probably need counselling too. To

come to terms with the fact that we could have a 50–50 chance with them. You are not going to walk away, work through the stage to when that child is ready to go. Stefan is not stupid, he is very bright. I used to think he is average because of having Down's, but he is a very very bright boy, and emotionally turned on because of what he has to live with. So he is completely aware of what is going on around him and I imagine he is going to realise that I am going to have . . . and my argument is, okay, if he is going to live with that thought, knowing he could get it, give him the chance to know whether he has got it or not. And . . . what is the point of him going to university? What I want is not what he would necessarily want. And the fact that . . . they are getting closer and they could come up . . . which I suppose is fair. I just feel that it should be a family decision. Okay, Louisa is too young to make the decision. Professor B., the Dr . . . He's like [imitating patronising tone]: "I know what you are going to say. I know what you want to talk about". But I just think that they are saying that it is for me. That it's what I want and not for the children. And they are probably right. But I don't see myself as the carer for maybe the rest of my life. Why shouldn't I know, you know? And it is probably again, completely selfish of me, talking to you about this . . . I can see that the whole situation so far as Stefan is concerned is just going to be taken out of my hands when he reaches eighteen. And I just object to the fact that I am here doing all the caring and everything . . .

MK: What happens when you present your case and you say that you would like to be able to prepare for things?

ID: To be quite frank some of the counselling, maybe it's because we have doubts, but some of it is just well . . . [agitated] I don't know, I just get frustrated, because I'm having to go and shout at people, and yell at people [to be heard]. I don't know, perhaps I am not being reasonable. Perhaps I am being completely selfish [nervous laughter]. I don't know. You just come away from there thinking: what does it take? If I was a multi millionaire you would be up in the list by now, but because I can't afford to do this, you know. It would be interesting to see if we could afford to do it, what would happen. It worries me because I just feel that the whole situation is completely out of our control, and we are just here waiting for them to come up with something.

Such conflicts of interest and mixed loyalties evoke the concerns and feelings of helplessness experienced by numerous in-marrying partners who find themselves positioned as long-term carers, possibly for multiple family members and across the generations. In this moving testimony, Isobel's plea for 'juvenile genetic testing' is bounced back rhetorically through her questioning of the medical profession's accountability: 'what right is it of them to decide?' (cf. Laurie Williams, Chapter 5). She is arguing that genetic counsellors should be educated to understand what couples desire in childrearing and how a disabling condition affects their hopes and expectations of parenthood. Patients, in other words, are perfectly able to inform and educate professionals. Again, it is surely significant that a study of public attitudes in Britain on aspects of genetic testing elicited an overwhelming response in favour of granting parents the right to ask for their child to be tested for genetic disorders that develop in adulthood (Human Genetics Commission 2001:58). While this may be the majority view of adults and parents, as earlier case material has shown, young adults – including those who have been fortunate to receive favourable results – are wary about letting younger siblings experience the same testing experiences they have been through (see Kingston/Richardson family, Chapter 5). In addition, it is possible that in some situations people may try to have children genetically tested without their express consent and non-consensual testing may potentially be facilitated by the availability of 'direct' genetic tests supplied over-the-counter or via the Internet (Human Genetics Commission 2003, 2002). Seeing the larger picture, then, genetic testing may confound all 'experts' – professionals and non-professionals alike, since there are no necessarily right or wrong ways to proceed. So far as Isobel's case is concerned, her question begs as a response the way that claims over rights, as ethically sanctioned legal positions, refer to quite different beliefs about care of the self as 'social anatomy' and forms of moral agency. One ongoing dilemma for the Daley family relates to the problem of making links between disease causality and attribution. Isobel is uncertain how to distinguish between what in her son is currently manifest as Down' syndrome and what may possibly turn out to be HD. Does the Down's mask the HD, or is part of the Down's behaviour already mixed up in the symptomatology of progressive deterioration? Her insistence that 'I should be able to prepare what I want for him . . . Down's children also age more quickly than other children' is also an admission – an alternative confession – of embodied foreknowledge as prophylactic agency.[17] The 'growth' of Isobel's children depends on what she activates as knowledge about them and the kinds of pre-emptive relations that this knowledge temporally anticipates (cf. McCallum 1996; Sam McDonald, Chapter 3).[18]

What can be seen as a particular explanatory model of 'pre-emptive' rationality transforms kinship into the active temporality of pragmatic preparation work. It is necessary for the Daley family to calculate the children's future probable health against the costs of a mortgage, insurance, upkeep of a home, a university education, and so on. Those who live the kinship consequences of the new technology know that the making of pre-symptomatic persons requires preparation, and in this sense there can be absolutely nothing 'natural' about a genetic 'predisposition' to a certain late-onset illness. This is the long story of why Isobel regrets her earlier disinterest in prenatal exclusion testing and how forms of stratification and kin equivalence may co-exist in subtle and contradictory ways as 'discrimination' within such affected families. Would it not be reasonable to ask in the same breath: How many parents who have not needed recourse to assisted reproductive or genetic technology harbour similar predispositions to stratified care-giving and affection, but would be less ready to confront or acknowledge these feelings?

Summary: the 'new genetic family'

This chapter has shown how a positively diagnosed pre-symptomatic mother of three 'at risk' children and an in-marrying carer of a symptomatic husband with two 'at risk' children strive each in their own way to limit the interventions associated with further technological innovation in human reproductive genetics. Further, these case study examples have begun to illuminate some of the multi-faceted and contradictory aspects of pre-symptomatic family life that have remained up to now largely hidden as private or unarticulated testimonies, eclipsed from broader public debate and commentary. Specifically, the analysis has exposed how little is known about the way couples make reproductive choices when one partner is affected or will be affected with a hereditary condition, and how former reproductive decisions may rebound on future family life and ideas about relatedness. It will be crucial for further policy ethnography and analysis in this area to address the ways family planning takes place as the sharing of reproductive dilemmas, and how this involves exchanges of information over time between kin, not only prior to, but long after the birth event.

Directly caught up in the midst of clinical dilemmas and difficult reproductive decision-making, the desire of parents to protect potential offspring from serious genetic conditions is a powerful *raison d'etre* for developing further innovations in preconception diagnostics. Many would not deny the amelioration of human suffering exerts a powerful pull, at least for the majority perspective. Clinicians, scientists, patients and policy-makers may thus be surprised and confounded by seemingly counter-intuitive ideas and sensibilities. Clearly some women undergoing prenatal testing *do* want to keep an affected baby, not because all the doubts, reservations, fears, worries and anticipated hardships cannot be removed or resolved, but because they do not want the decision to have been made on account of the knowledge that advanced technology brings. Being tested, wanting more information and excluding non-knowledge does not necessarily always lead to acting on such insight. Finding out about the genetic status of the IVF embryo prior to transfer and uterine implantation may be sufficient knowledge in itself for some mothers and couples. As I noted in Chapter 3, it may be that those with the strongest kin connections feel impelled 'to care not to know', and thus not to generate new diagnostic and prognostic information for others, through intuiting the meaning of saying nothing. How widely spread these sentiments travel across families, we do not as yet know for want of existing empirical studies.[19] Nonetheless these are certainly issues to which future public health communication and risk management initiatives will need to be sensitive, especially so in the framing of genetic education campaigns for clinicians and health-allied practitioners.

Linked to this, we have seen that prenatal exclusion testing and pre-implantation genetic diagnosis open up new categories of ethical consciousness and notions of parental responsibility. I have suggested social critiques can start to analyse these shifts in terms of the way people frame issues about the cultural burdens of elimination and how such accounts get narrated through highly intimate languages. These narrative discourses are fruitful to explore for several reasons. Describing forms of social resistance may be impeded by the absence of an easily accessible or culturally sanctioned vocabulary. Daisy and Isobel both castigate themselves as 'selfish', attributes they imagine others might use, but clearly their views do not fit with the conventional sociobiological notion of selfish genes as autonomous replicators devoid of moral agency. More profoundly still for considerations of public policy and welfare debates, genetic testing technology raises the scenario of mothers, fathers and grandparents realising that they do not always know how best to parent 'at risk' children. There is continuing concern that parents are morally culpable and 'responsible' for having transmitted a genetic susceptibility of which they had no prior knowledge or, in certain cases, which they actively denied or withheld from disclosure. What we can see emerging, then, is the attempt by 'at risk', confirmed pre-symptomatic and currently symptomatic parents to talk through an unfamiliar and highly intimate range of kinship relationality whose emotional parameters may at times be negotiated and redefined as new moral knowledge. This can be taken as just one representation of the 'new genetic family'. In these contexts, this becomes evident as a composite of persons who know each other in relation to their own articulated management of genetic information and genetically acquired moral dilemmas.

When we analyse the temporal embeddedness of exclusion as conflicts of interest between such divergent kin, it is evident that the terms of reference informing local familial discourses are not themselves underscored by an overriding preoccupation with biomedical concepts of risk probability. Within families, kinship ethics may unfold as anticipatory forms of sibling equivalence, for example, and notions of endebted risk may be morally inflected in terms of notions of relative degrees of (dis)loyalty. Putting these notions to work, or rather seeing them enacted in practice, may show up how new genetic families appear both to fragment along lines of divisiveness (see Chapters 3–5), as well as how they cohere – perhaps more surprisingly – through novel idioms of inclusiveness. Understanding the nature of these differences may become the ideological basis for expressing and channelling what in time may come to be seen as new moral sentiments of 'tradition' (cf. Dolgin 2000; Finkler 2000). In the light of existing cultural critiques of biological reductionism and gene fetishism, it is clear there is an urgent need to separate out the geneticisation of medical and popular discourse from the more uncertain and affectively charged kinship talk of social anatomy. Our case material has painted an early picture as to how such local idioms make up the subjective experience of a quotidian, everyday genetics. Instead of hearing technical and impersonal genetic information about the role of genes, proteins, cells, nuclei and chromosomes, indigenous accounts are built up through ambivalence in terms of notions of time, relationships, relatedness, uncertainty, predictive knowledge, death and uncertain reproduction. In terms of future genetic health policy, a strong focus on culture as forms of resistance – in particular attentiveness to embodiment narratives as critical reflections on temporality and relatedness – can be fruitful in paving the way toward more sensitive clinical practice in the area of client decision-making and reproductive 'choice'. Thus we have seen how the refiguring of relations through a relational ethics challenges the conventional orthodoxy of bioethical 'first' principles – the norms of autonomy, beneficence, non-maleficence and justice/obligations of fairness – and may on occasion even disrupt familiar expressions of love and emotion as the 'natural' sentiments of parenthood. These findings are of anthropological and sociological relevance in their own right, but they contribute more broadly of course to debates about public understandings of genetic science, public trust in medical expertise and public attitudes to regulation.

7

Concluding remarks

Predictive medicine is a complex art

More often than not, predictive testing technology relies on the power of imagination. Interpreting and imparting to others the meaning of genetic information, or even withholding information, are acts that almost always involve the transfer of emotion between persons. Communicating probabilities and results through empathetic understanding, or living one's future in the face of new prognostic knowledge – in one way or another predictive medicine makes us 'see' ourselves in a different light. Unexpected health information may be interpreted in certain instances as helpful for a particular individual; on other occasions there may be unwelcome or even shocking news. Whatever the specific test outcome, enhancing predictability in human genomics produces the inescapable irony one may never know in advance quite how any given testee will respond. The art of predictive medicine is characterised by the richness of contingency and conjecture that is the human condition.

Of course there is the science of prediction too. Scientific knowledge inheres in the proven capacity of research geneticists, molecular biologists and bioinformaticians to identify links between specific genes, or clusters of genes, and particular diseases. But even these searches for correlation may be subject to uncertainty and imprecision. Within the clinical genetics community, it is a practically undisputed claim that the presence of multiple predisposing variants in several genes may make the ongoing search for links with disease challenging to study. In fact, many scientists today acknowledge that genes may turn out to be fairly poor predictors of complex diseases. Aside from monogenic conditions caused by changes in a single gene, there is still considerable uncertainty about the role of genes and the environment in the progression of so-called common complex diseases. The term 'complex disease' applies to most major afflictions of the Western world and describes conditions like cancer, cardiovascular disease, obesity, dementias or arthritis that develop as a result of the interaction between genetic and non-biological factors (e.g. lifestyle factors such as diet, smoking, exercise, exposure to pollution). In the cases of heart disease and cancer, for example, many different genetic mutations in several different genes may each play a minor role, and a single genetic trait may predispose to one disease whilst being protective of another. In addition, multiple environmental factors may often play a more formative role in disease development than genetic make-up itself. This variability towards disease susceptibility makes it difficult for tests to predict precisely the likelihood one will become ill. For multifactorial diseases in the wider population, predictive genetic testing cannot provide any assurances: all that can be indicated is a likely susceptibility for a specific tested condition with no certainty of the associated illness developing.

As more tests for genetic susceptibility and 'predisposition profiling' are researched and developed by pharmaceutical and biotechnology companies, genetic health service providers will face huge infrastructural and procedural challenges. Genetic counsellors and other health practitioners will need to acquire specific skills and training in the art of listening, interpreting and explaining highly uncertain risk predictions to the large proportion of the population likely to be identified as susceptible to common complex diseases. Working out what counts as adequate counselling care and then providing integrated services so that each presenting individual can access these facilities according to their own specific needs will not be limited to the work of specialist NHS genetic clinics alone. As current government proposals in Britain suggest, this provision will fall increasingly to professional multidisciplinary teams and especially to new working collaborations within the primary healthcare field where the general practitioner is expected to play a crucial informative role. The creation of new genetic 'facts' and the imparting of complex and possibly indeterminate risk quantification require therefore an enhanced medical workforce skilled in the subtle art of human communication for future medicines management.

Discerning the clinical validity and utility of different tests will be another important facet of this 'humanities-science' interface in genetics. As global pharmaceutical companies seek to expand their markets, and as the growing commercialisation of genetic tests brings predictive knowledge sooner or later to the interested home user, there is considerable concern certain tests may be deployed because they are seen to be 'new' and 'fashionable' rather than useful and relevant. Tests that are introduced without appropriate clinical evaluation could exacerbate a heightened wave of medicalisation rather than facilitate improved patient care (Melzer and Zimmern 2002). Developing good practice among the clinical genetics community depends, in part, on the ability to discriminate between tests with so-called high 'informational impact' that demand a higher standard of analytic verification than low informational tests because they are expected to yield 'significant health outcomes' (Human Genetics Commission 2003:58). Gauging the 'delicate balance in the 'risk-benefit' of genetic tests will be an important review function of the UK Genetic Testing Network not least since the more predictive tests an individual under-goes, the likelier it is that some tests will turn out as 'false negatives' or 'false positives' (Levitt 1999).[1] It is not inconceivable that the entire rationale of pre-dictive medicine – namely the intended benefits of a healthier population that is more cost-effective to manage – could be undone by such inaccuracies. With false negatives, genetic misinformation may cultivate a false sense of reassur-ance in the tested person whose sense of 'genetic untouchability' may lead to less healthy or unhealthy lifestyle pursuits. There may be the popular misun-derstanding that 'good genes' means one can indulge without consequence in a fat-rich diet, for example. Alternatively one may ignore certain symptoms or delay seeking medical advice. 'False positives', on the other hand, may lead to an unnecessary sense of worry in the testee who may fear he or she is at risk of developing an illness, whilst in fact there is no actual scientific basis for genetic predisposition. For some, this foreknowledge of an illness whose symptoms are yet-to-be-made-visible may lead to a sense of 'genetic fatalism' characterised by the belief there is nothing one can do for oneself to prevent the course of a predicted future illness. Such is the suggestiveness of health information, it is not impossible some testees found to be 'false positive' could make themselves genuinely ill over their incessant worrying they may become ill.[2] These points simply offer examples as to how a potentially inexact science *may* encounter early teething problems, if not more durable obstacles, in real-ising *all* of its intended benefits in the so-called 'coming revolution in health care' (Department of Health 2003:1).

Contexts teach

If health professionals require ongoing training in the new genetics, consumer education in the new testing era will also intensify as state-sanctioned initiatives aim to inform the public about the different forms of predictive testing. In pledg-ing its commitment to the 'golden age of bio-science', the British government has observed the importance of 'increasing public understanding of genetics and ensuring public confidence through a robust and proportionate system of regu-lation' (Department of Health 2003:1, 23). Perhaps one of the most critical – or should one say civilising? – aspects of such health education campaigns will be the inclusion of users and patients on relevant research drafting boards and policy committees. It is not just a matter of professionals communicating genetic risk information *to* individuals or patients. Different publics versed in their own 'expert' knowledge beliefs must also be involved actively in educating policy makers if 'evidence-based care' is to have any formative influence in the evaluation of emerging initiatives, interventions and technologies.

Since genetic tests fall across such a wide spectrum of implication – ranging from the highly penetrant mutations to those with loose associations with disease and those that are of relatively little health consequence – the acquisition of a substantive empirical evidence base will take some time to establish. Future policy decisions need to be based on firm evidence about how individuals and families really do respond, not on assumptions about what people's reactions will be. While this book has examined the experiences of one patient population in Britain affected by a single-gene condition, the case material presented here has a far wider relevance beyond the predicament of Huntington's Disease (HD) alone. Though obviously not everyone who goes for predictive testing stands to lose or gain as much from the news that an HD test can reveal, one can extrapolate in certain limited ways from the decision-making dilemmas of individuals and families analysed during the course of this ethnographic exercise. When faced with the realisation kin and kith (i.e. blood and non-blood relatives) stood to inherit the symptoms of this illness, participants in my research recounted a number of personal and interpersonal difficulties whose effects could span numerous years or even across the generations. Their deeply intimate testimonies describe some of the dilemmas associated with emerging regimes of predispositional truth that redefine concepts of health, illness and normality through the reclassification of persons as 'pre-ill' or 'pre-symptomatic'. The sense of confusion experienced by self-identified 'genetic escapees', the mixed sentiments aroused by conflicting loyalties within families, the subtle shift in kinship allegiances between siblings, between parents and offspring, or between affines give expression to new familial idioms of inclusiveness, belonging, sharing, discrimination and exclusion. The multi-faceted nature of these perceived obligations confounds notions of relationality as much as they make and re-invent the terms by which kin imagine they can get on and get by with one another. There is absolutely nothing predictable about these imaginings: the genetic tie can make or break relations. Genes, in other words, can be the indexical symbol of surprise.

We learn additionally from these important narratives that the acquisition of genetic knowledge can bring with it an unacceptable degree of anxiety about the future, particularly where there is no therapeutic treatment available. The institutional hiatus that falls between the time of diagnosis and therapeutic intervention opens up what we can identify as the 'the prognostic gap'. This gap is both a moral, socio-political expanse and one that is embodied as the lived experiential gap of subjective chronicity, deep uncertainty and anticipation (see Chapter 3). Through their evasions or non-disclosures, my research interlocutors illustrate too that the fact of having more genetic knowledge about oneself or a loved one does not necessarily mean one knows how best to act on that knowledge. As they explain in their own words, there are no necessarily pre-given ethical formulas or principles by which 'correct' decisions can be reached in certain applied situations. One arrives at ethics a bit like one arrives at kinship: one learns to get by. Contexts teach!

A further extrapolation comes from the observation one might actively choose not to know potentially exacting information about one's genes. In fact preferring not to know details of one's biological heredity may characterise a greater extent of the populace than might be commonly anticipated at the present time. Low uptake of predictive genetic tests may not be confined simply to those affected by autosomal dominant conditions, as has been found to be the case for the HD population. Turning away from this kind of predictive knowledge may turn out to be the express preference of widely diverse sectors of society including (say) certain ethnic or religious groups, particular age cohorts such as the elderly, the well educated, or disadvantaged poor. These more cautious or reluctant populations display indisposition; they are in a manner of speaking the 'indisposed'. Public health genetics, meanwhile, might be moving towards a more enthusiastic uptake of genetic delivery systems such that we may soon reach a situation where individuals are seen as irresponsible for not undergoing genetic tests where these are available. A number of my research participants have telling things to say on such matters of choice and intention. Certain of their statements indicate that mechanisms are needed to protect individuals from misleading claims based on the widely held perception of the predictiveness of genetics (cf. Crossley 1996). The advertising of newly commercialised 'predisposition' tests may provoke a range of feelings amongst the public ranging from unease, anxiety, curiosity and uncertainty. In the worst case scenario, biotechnology activists and others already see parallels between the aggressive promotion of genetic tests by pharmaceutical companies and the psychological exploitation of individuals unleashed as the 'marketing of fear', all in the name of bio-industrial profit (Moynihan *et al.* 2002). Consumer education in genetics needs then to include in its remit a healthy component of scepticism. As actor Woody Allen once said: 'I have seen the future, and it is very much like the present, only longer'.

(The myth of) pre-emptive individualism

Scepticism, however, may not always be the natural ally of health education regimes that promote the ideal of good health as an individual responsibility, even a civic duty and project for the self to 'work on'. In the era of predictive bioscience and biomedicine, the discourse of the 'healthy citizen', as the cultivation of a Foucauldian type of technology of the self – a late-industrial form of modern subjectivity – is sustained by a number of intersecting moral claims, appeals and requirements. Essentially these depend on buttressing individual interest in ideologies of individualism, the individual's 'right to self-determination' and notions of self-reliance, for instance, alongside political ideologies that stress measures of efficiency in healthcare. On the one hand there is the rise of pharmacogenetics research with its promise of tailor-made medicines as well as the prospect of personalised and affordable DNA profiles for everyone at some point in the future (see Chapter 1). At the same time, existing NHS plans in Britain are already designed around the concept of patient pledges and the commitment to lead healthy lifestyles. New patient-GP 'contracts', it is envisaged, will be signed documents imbued with moral sanction. A patient may have to agree to give up junk food, say, in return for care for high cholesterol or other health problems. In brief, what this may mean is that overweight patients will have to diet before they become eligible to see their GP (Macintyre 2003). Now since general practitioners will play increasingly key roles in information communication relating to genetic health, as mentioned above, these 'responsibility pledges' are already forerunners to the making of 'new genetic citizens', a term applied with critical precision by Alan Petersen and Robin Bunton (2002: 180–207). Moreover, the ideal of 'working on oneself' to produce an efficient and adaptable subject is apparent in the pre-emptive rationality that says greater patient awareness of illness leads to improved self-help, which in turn will save on public health expenditure. Many people are not responding with scepticism; rather they are buying into this vision, literally consuming it. Witness the lightning growth of the self-diagnostics market. A recent report for the market analyst Mintel found that British consumers currently spend £55 million a year on self-diagnostic devices such as blood pressure monitors, pregnancy tests, ovulation kits, body-fat monitors, tests for blood cholesterol, peak flow meters and blood glucose monitors used by diabetics (Hawkes 2003). Compared to the indisposed, self-diagnosticians can be co-opted potentially that much more readily by genetic regimes of pre-dispositional profiling so as to fit the desired model of the responsible health-seeking citizen. All such methods of co-optation, as strategies of geneticisation, enhance rationalities of 'pre-emptive individualism'. Pre-emptive individualism is a form of political hegemony dependent on

the strategic manipulation of already-written futures. It features both within
and beyond the domain of genetic reification so that the late modernist can
speak reasonably of encompassing pre-emptive cultures. Consider the already
written futures contained in debt-repayment systems (capitalist futures tied to
loan schemes); the already written futures contained in the pre-emptive offen-
sive strikes of states' foreign policy moves (international war machines); or the
already written futures of educational selection systems. (University Student
Admissions Committees be warned. Apparently it is now possible to identify
children with the potential to go to university by the age of 3! [see Utley 2003].)[3]

Exposing the precarious nature of these rhetorical strategic ploys and discursive associations is one of the counter-intuitive arguments of this book. Look
closely and contained in the ethnographic chapters is the myth of pre-emptive
individualism. We can see from the narratives presented (Chapters 3–6), that
many of the ethical dilemmas opened up by the applications of biotechnology
offer also ironically the opportunity to re-think and re-theorise human genetics
as a social critique of Western individualism. Discerning the tension that inheres
in the increasingly personalised and increasingly relational nature of genetic
information is one clue. Let me break this down into two summary parts: (1) the
claims of interdependent persons; and (2) making claims about interdependent
information.

Interdependent persons

While the expansion of public genetic services will drive medical provision
for much of the Western world in the coming years, clinical space is not the
only arena where genetic dilemmas assume explicit prominence. The question
of what health information is transmitted in and through the medium of an
'anticipated prognosis' can no longer be limited to the exclusive domain of
the medical practitioner, understood as the professional's acts of 'inward' and
'outward' prognostication, of foreseeing and foretelling respectively (Christakis
1999:192–4, see Chapters 3 and 4). Bioethical debates relevant to the clinician
concerning the ethics of 'unsolicited' information disclosure to family members
(and other agencies) need to be apprehended in terms of the complications
of disclosure practices that reach far beyond the space of the genetics clinic.
Visions of 'one-stop shops' for diagnostic health or 'gene boutiques' set up
as franchises within sports shops or health clubs, for example, will employ a
new brigade of 'medical' professionals such as 'lifestyle health instructors',
dieticians and complementary therapists. If lifestyle advice based on genetic
test results will be offered to the public as 'privatised' genetic information
that does not belong to the state – since it potentially escapes the medical

records system of a National Health Service – there will be nothing, however, to stop such information being 'sold off' to other commercial companies. The privatisation of genetic surveillance may target 'at risk' individuals with direct-market vitamin supplements and medication, but without adequate regulation there are no enforceable sanctions legitimating the cultural question: whose social property is one's body?

Because genetic information is not simply information about an individual person but necessarily reveals knowledge about one's biological relations, the new genetics can be said to *literalise* kinship as webs of biological relatedness (cf. Finkler 2000 on the medicalisation of kinship). The narratives explored in the book show how the literalisation of kinship opens up a fresh discursive space for the cultural recognition of heredity as *social anatomies of interdependence*. These 'anatomies' present a direct challenge to the individualistic premises of gene fetishism and 'gene fatalism'. As several chapters have discussed, people may attempt to redefine hope and 'test out' misfortune in ways that necessarily implicate their next of kin. The 'facts' of heredity can no longer be construed as simply the traces of past biological transmission and what you can see ('traits' in oneself and others as comparative likeness), but arise as moral choices – or ethno-ethical knowledge – that shape personhood as future action. Heredity is what one decides to tell and how knowledge is shared; it is *made lively* as social anatomies of interdependence (Chapters 5 and 6).

We saw too that people's decision-making over whether to access what mainstream biomedical discourse constructs as the genetic 'truth' about themselves, and whether and how to tell such 'truth' to others, is a fascinating anthropological question concerning kinship temporality. When applications of genetic science become decisions about whether or not to get oneself tested, the shift from genes as simply pre-coded sets of instructions to the creation of pre-symptomatic information as certain foreknowledge about persons, needs to be understood as the process of anticipatory value reckoning. Understanding new temporal relations of embodiment and knowledge is, however, not confined to the case of HD or other late-onset conditions for which there is still no effective cure. Conceptualising issues of temporality has a far broader applicability to many of the clinical, research and socio-political operations of the new medical technologies. For example, biobanking and the circulations of bodily specimens through bio-archival space, the effects of temporal reversibility occasioned by stem cell technologies, the altered generational 'timelines' represented by cloned entities, the bio-economic rationales of pre-emptively 'underwriting' persons in health insurance. We have seen further that detailed analysis of the ways people embody the genetics of kinship temporality as practices of 'genealogical ethics' shows up why genetic information can be

considered unique and different from other categories of medical information. Several of the chapters have shown that recognition of this uniqueness
does not, however, *necessarily* support essentialist attributions of the gene
as 'ur-thing', or the social proliferation of 'hypergenetic ideologies', to borrow cultural theorist and biologist Donna Haraway's expression (2000:89–
95; cf. Murray 1997 on 'genetic exceptionalism'). Furthermore, getting to the
heart of people's decision-making in these familial spaces – namely to moral
spaces outside the medical context of the clinic – allows us to challenge further the conventional assumption that more genetic information in itself will
create more choice for individuals. If genetic information does not necessarily
create more choice, how do we shape our critical enquiries about predictive
medicine futures? How do we contemplate what it means to see the future as
an age of personalised DNA sequencing and how do we ask what this would
mean for the ordinary person? How do we evaluate the idea we stand to live
longer, healthier and happier lives?

Interdependent information

At another level, the social proliferation of genetic health information invites
us to think about post-genomic sociality as the cultural ordering of interdependent information. It is not necessary to look into the distance to see why this
is politically meaningful. New genetic knowledge already elicits cultural value
as the process of making complex cross-links. Technologies such as the DNA
chip – which many scientists claim will be able to scan an individual patient,
read one's genetic make-up in detail, and detect abnormal or malfunctioning
genes – highlight the possibilities deriving from the union of genes and com-
puters. This merging of genetic and digital technologies, the coming together of
the information sciences and the life sciences, promises to shift us fast forward
into the era of a *systematised* predictive medicine. The point I want to underscore is that there need be nothing strictly inevitable or predetermined about
such 'predictive' trajectories. Indeed what is taken for the systematic can come
together in quite strange and unpredictable ways. True, chip technology will
mean that the results of a whole range of tests can be brought together into a
single assessment or risk.[4] For those technologically advanced social systems
and economies that can buy into the R&D innovation base, this might sound or
look beautifully simple. But what can appear as reductionism or cost-efficiency
rationales must also be seen as processes that depend on the intertwining of
complex calculations, histories and futures.

Take the field that is known as systems biology. Systems biology aims to provide a rigorous knowledge base for the complex network of processes that we

call 'Life'. But many practitioners in the field know that deep epistemological growth depends on dynamic collaborations across the different disciplines. If future expert knowledge depends on the forging and maintenance of complex links within and between disciplines, there is nothing particularly straightforward about this. Developments in the domain of genomics and proteonomics, advances in informatics and complex modelling, the growing interest of physicists in living systems and developments in disciplines as far apart as molecular genetics, experimental medicine, mathematics, neuroscience, physiology and analytical chemistry face the challenge of interdisciplinary integration if they are to incorporate all processes of the living cell in a dynamic description. Precisely such an experiment in the informational modelling of cross-linkage is how we might characterise the contemporary emergence of DNA databanks for health research purposes. So-called 'biobanks' are centralised repositories of disparate (health) information. As material artefacts built up through the epidemiological and socio-cultural architecture of processual cross-linkage, they are informational designs of a particular kind.[5] But to build the architecture, people must agree to participate actively in such construction work, both to the object itself that is 'biobank' and to the guiding vision that underpins it. Members of the public must *be* the building blocs, as it were, giving of their support in the hope that knowledge about the links between genes and disease will be inferred from the systematic collection, storage and interpretation of recruits' donated genetic samples and related social data.[6] Genetic donors thus buy into an expectation, namely a social vision of improved health for the collectivity, even if they may not be the direct beneficiaries of the resultant accumulating medical knowledge. Such projects depend fundamentally on the production and management of cross-correlated knowledge. Highly disparate and anonymised data will be transformed into aggregate information – a synthesis of sorts. 'A unified information system' that can link across different data sets to establish points of interconnectivity was the House of Lords' (2001: 6.25) chosen description.[7] Underpinning these practices of inter-linkage is the assumption that persons, via their stored samples and bio-data, can be 'traced' over time – in the case of UK Biobank, at least over the next decade (2003–2013). For without the longitudinal factor, research interconnectivity has no prospect. Scientists, epidemiologists, health administrators and others must therefore model interconnective knowledge production on another socially robust model of knowledge: namely, the making explicit of consent agreements that members of the public will have to give prior to taking part in such information experiments.

What then to make of the UK government's Genetics White Paper? This puts forward the possibility of screening all babies at birth and storing information about their genetic profile for future use in tailoring healthcare according to their needs.[8] Where the Department of Health (2003:44–45) describes this plan in terms of the production of a 'comprehensive map of their [new-born babies] key genetic markers, or even their entire genome', a sceptic might see this as a surreptitious 'biobanking' exercise for neonates. In line with current investments in NHS information technology, the baby's genetic information could be entered at birth on their electronic patient record for future biomedical use and health monitoring.[9] As the cynic would say, genetic surveillance creeps into the lifeline at the earliest possible chance. But issues of data privacy, confidentiality and consent with regard to genetic information collection and its applications must be central to all cross-linkage data projects (see Human Genetics Commission 2002). As mentioned, a key debate in the literature often tied to notions of the informed subject and ideals of active citizenship, is the right of the person as well as blood kin to know genetic information about oneself. Increasingly important in the future, though currently not enshrined in current British statute, is the right of the subject not to know, or to refuse to know, genetic information about oneself (see Chapter 4).[10] Of course newborn babies clearly cannot be asked for their informational consent. Striking to note then that the aforementioned White Paper on genetics was silent on this – quite simply the issue did not appear as an explicit social and ethical problem. Rather it was presumed that babies at birth could be or will be 'recruited' as informational subjects into such programmes. Of course one doesn't have to stretch the imagination to see how in practical terms this will happen. It will be parents who will be asked to give their consent on behalf of their children, and this consent will be routinised or 'normalised' by practitioners in the name of the baby's future good health. Much in the manner that existing screening programmes for newborns are justified for phenylketonuria and congenital hypothyroidism, things will all appear simple, safe and sanitised. The kind of genetic knowledge we want to embrace or refuse, and subsequently the kind of genetic futures we will inhabit – such genetic worlds can be referenced and signalled by way of multiple informatic connections and cross-linkages. It matters then how we rationalise in cultural terms the bringing together of different sources of genetic knowledge. Similarly it matters how we insist on keeping strands of data apart. If chip technology means the results of a whole range of tests can be brought together or standardised into a single assessment or 'risk' profile, what then of excluding certain information? What of keeping interdependent knowledge apart? Because the development of such tests might make it difficult to focus on specific chromosomal sites, at the very least a particular consent issue arises. What if one wants to be genetically tested for a specific condition, to have susceptibility, predictive or diagnostic testing performed in a limited way? People may be informed of risks that they didn't want to know about without prior in-depth counselling or advice. For example, an increased risk of susceptibility to Alzheimer's disease has been associated with one of the genes comprising the Genovations 'Cardio' genetic test marketed by the US company Great Smokies Diagnostics Laboratory.[11] But what if one doesn't want to know in advance everything about one's genome? And if therapeutic interventions are not available, how is one to act in any case on such foreknowledge? How useful and how pre-disposing to human happiness is such knowledge? (see Chapters 3–6). Or could it be that by the time gene chip technology arrives we will have moved towards a situation of mandatory testing? Imagine if health costs become so exorbitant that a government calls for compulsory testing for genetic diseases or refuses to pay the health costs for a baby whose genetic disease would have been preventable had it been tested? Will it be the case that parents one day will be seen as irresponsible if they have children without genetic testing?

We are at a critical time. We possess the science and technology to make everyone more standard, or to create a world for the first time where we can hope to understand, appreciate, respect and celebrate the diversity of difference. While prenatal screening or testing and pre-implantation genetic diagnosis may be worthwhile and beneficial in certain cases, at the same time the proliferation of 'reprogenetic' technologies can contribute to a heightened medicalisation of pregnancy through pressures to abort after diagnoses of disability, or through the selection of non-genetically vulnerable embryos for uterine implantation. As pre-emptive cultures medicalise kin relations and fundamentally redefine our conceptions of health, well being and personhood in the age of new genetic rationalism, whether or not one becomes 'pre-symptomatic' will increasingly preoccupy not just the living but those yet to be born. Attaching the term 'designer babies' or 'made to order' babies in blanket fashion to all preconception technologies skews debate. Different concepts of inclusion and exclusion inform the practice of 'selecting out' traits – the deployment of genetic testing for medical reasons – as we saw in Chapters 5 and 6. 'Selecting in' traits so that genetic enhancement is pursued as an ideal of perfectibility for non-medical reasons, is a different form of consumerist selection that entangles the increasingly personalised with the increasingly standardised (Konrad 2004). As the standardisation, differentiation and specialisation of genetic knowledge become more and more obvious as inter-linked projects, so complementary and contradictory effects are generated. And as cross-linkage is facilitated through 'informational expansion' (e.g., the method of activating longitudinal intervention frames) and 'informational contraction' (the conceptual refinement of issues of data privacy, confidentiality, consent agreements), we would do well not to lose sight of the importance of protections against unfair discrimination.

Linked to this is the urgent need to refine our concepts of genetic privacy and to see these enshrined in new genetic privacy legislation. Interdisciplinary collaborations between human rights lawyers, social anthropologists and sociologists, scientists and ethicists, among others, are required to address these regulatory issues and their specific application in both national and international settings.[12]

Linkage by translocation

Just as systems biology depends on integrative analysis for a dynamic description of the living cell, so the humanities and social sciences may find fruitful points of theoretical convergence between disciplines, as well as in partnership with the biosciences, for re-describing the meanings and attributes of 'life' in biosocial context. *Narrating the New Predictive Genetics* has attempted a synthetic study of 'cross-talking' value by using the descriptive tool and metaphor of ethnography as linkage map (Chapters 1 and 2; 3–6). Borrowing a biological idiom from classical genetics theory, I have undertaken a series of ethnographic and conceptual 'translocations' in order to introduce the translocated role of the anthropologist/diviner. The ethnographer's immersion in the practical realities of 'everyday genetics' has been used as the key tool or 'technique' for the facilitation of moves between discrete areas – both locales and subject thematics – so as to assert provisional linkages between the fields of bioscience, anthropology and bioethics.

One aim has been to arrive at a broadened definition of bioethics beyond the taxonomy of rules, regulations and principles that characterise traditional 'normative' or meta-ethical approaches. Bringing together bioethics and bioethnography for rich contextualisation, our analysis has illustrated how moral reasoning, as processes of engagement, can be valued within situated research practice and theoretical reflexivity. I have sought to clarify, in addition, how current anthropological work on kinship and morality can contribute to contemporary concerns in medical science, health policy and constructions of genetic personhood outside of the conceptual framework designated by mainstream 'bioethics'. Via such modified translocation work, the viability of an ethno-ethics of divination and prophetic power has been approached in terms of a 'relational ethics' that explores local moralities of information revelation and knowledge disclosure between kin. As part of this argument I have wanted to show how social anthropology can add an important cross-cultural dimension to certain contemporary genomics and society debates. The pivot of comparative focus is not a cross-cultural genetics as such, but the processes by which flows of information engender cultural value as forms of moral agency, relational or embodied personhood. The reader will find references to a wide-ranging literature covering Eastern Uganda, Nigeria, Amazonia, Indonesia, Papua New Guinea, North India. Extrapolating from these translocations, we can carry across to other contexts the observation that terms such as 'health', 'normality' and 'disability' are not objective and universal definitions across time and place. The different cultural meanings attached to notions of pre-emption, prediction and the pre-symptomatic will change and shift over time, and similarly different individuals, families and kin relations are likely to inflect these terms with their own set of values or core symbols. Beware! Pre-emptive individualism may not be as stabile an ideology as it seems at first blush.

In sum, prognosticating a person's health through prophetic genetics can never be simply a matter of 'revealing' genetic knowledge as an 'objective' scientific diagnosis about chromosomal alignments. It is never simply a matter of 'reading off' genetic markers and correlating linkages between alleles. Approaches from anthropology have a lot to say about how various categories of genetic information come to be transferred between different social bodies, and how such information engenders cultural value as certain paradoxes. Relaying such findings to interested anthropologists is one thing, but increasingly anthropology finds itself being called upon to count in ways that exceed conventional disciplinary boundaries. Seeking actively to create sites of potential collaboration with clinical geneticists, health professionals and bioethicists, is all part of the ongoing task of seeking to 'translocate' culture across and between various biosocial domains.

Appendix

This research deployed a variety of methods, including open-ended, semi-structured interviews with Huntington's affected individuals (from twenty-four families); more structured conversational enquiries with members of relevant user groups and health professionals; the collection of medical genealogies for most families together with other primary data; and participant observation. Each of these is discussed below.

In-depth and semi-structured home-based interviews were conducted with families from different parts of the UK (North, Midlands, South, Scotland, Wales and Northern Ireland). Adult interviewees were typically white Caucasian, heterosexual, middle class, Christian (Protestant). Research participants were interviewed individually, and where appropriate, as part of a family group or as a couple. One important aim of the study was to include as many consenting members of each contacted family as possible, including wherever possible data collection across the generations. In some cases, it was possible to record up to four generations within a given family. As a result those persons directly affected by the disease, as well as potential, current or ex-carers became the focus of the research. The average length of the interviews was between 3–5 hours. The interviews were usually tape-recorded sessions and were transcribed for further analysis.

Great care has been taken during the course of this study to ensure ethical practice, informed consent and confidentiality for the research. Confidentiality has been respected at all times during this project and will continue to be respected given the potentially discriminating effects of genetic information. All research participants were self-selecting at all stages of the research and interviews were only arranged with persons who consented to take part in the study and who understood and agreed with the study's aims and objectives. There is often a huge degree of secrecy between kin (especially siblings) regarding the sharing of genetic test results. Research participants have been reassured that the personal information collected during this study is to be used for research purposes only and shall not be divulged to any interested parties. All participants are protected by pseudonyms in the writing up of the research.

A range of topics were covered during the interviews including for example:

Notions of health, disease and illness and their relevance to genome research; local understandings of 'predictive' knowledge and notions of pre-emption; perceptions of risk and 'at risk' status; genetic information sharing within families and across the generations; ideas about the effect of genetic medicines and technology on biological inheritance; reproductive strategies and dilemmas (decision-making regarding prenatal diagnosis and pre-implantation diagnosis); experiences of accessing care and genetic counselling services; forms of patient activism within local user/community support HD groups. Data have been gathered from the following sub-groups.

(i) 'Pre-symptomatic' persons (e.g. offspring or siblings of HD diagnosed persons) who have not yet been tested themselves and are therefore known to be 'at risk' of developing the illness. This group includes those who are unsure whether to have the test sometime in the future as well as those who have decided against taking the test.

(ii) Those with a positive test result who are in the early onset stages of mental and physical decline ('early onset symptomatic').

(iii) Persons no longer 'at risk' due to their having obtained a positive (i.e. clear) test result.

(iv) Those married to 'at risk' or symptomatic persons. In-marrying partners were further distinguished by (i) gender and age, for example, as male/female or widow/widower; and present/future carer, (ii) those in-marrying partners who have knowledge of their partner's or an in-law's illness at the time of establishing a committed relationship.

(v) Offspring as descendants of an HD diagnosed person, and other first-degree relatives such as siblings, cousins, uncles, aunts, parents, grandparents. The research recruited a handful of cases of teenage offspring (usually around the age of 18–19 years) who stood potentially to implicate a parent (through an affected maternal or paternal line) in prospective illness through a positive test result.

Interview material has been supplemented by a variety of data including the diary extracts or personal notes recorded by research participants; several interviewees had drawn up family genealogies in the course of their own research investigations into medical family history. Some people had kept press clippings of HD or genetics-related events; others showed me obituary notices and family photos. This material is often highly personal and carries a strong emotional attachment for participants, and may also be intrinsically 'identifiable' to a particular named person. Care and sensitivity is required on the part of any researcher regarding the subsequent use of such materials, even when consent has been granted for their public dissemination. I have decided against the inclusion of any identifiable or visual materials that possibly might compromise interviewees' confidentiality, if not now, then in the future.

Besides the detailed work with the families there were three principal 'sites' for observation. These included:

(i) Going to meetings and discussion forums of local support groups for patients and carers; becoming acquainted with the news and activities taking place in the Huntington's community.

(ii) 'Sitting in' on a weekly basis on the genetic counselling sessions at the Clinical Genetics Unit of a London hospital for six months. Clinical practice, hospital protocol, patient-practitioner interaction was observed during certain 'clinic' days when patients attended pre-booked appointments or referrals seeking information and advice on diagnostic and predictive genetic testing.

(iii) Visits to the DNA laboratory of a hospital-based Molecular Genetics Division where staff were 'trailed' as much as possible in order that the research could understand better the scientific handling of DNA material and the various techniques for genetic testing.

In addition, a number of interviews and informal talks were conducted with various individuals. These included:

(i) Health professionals (consultant geneticists, genetic counsellors, embryologists, molecular biologists, consultant neuropsychiatrists) on medical genetics, professional roles and procedures, problems for practice and policy.

(ii) Information officers, regional care support advisors and local coordinators of user groups and various other support services/groups in the community advising on health, reproduction, family planning, and raising awareness about genetic conditions. Advice, collaboration and consultation with various user organisations has been very central to the research process, and a key factor in securing access to and acceptance within the Huntington's community at the outset of the study.

This book has focused on the experiences of six families in order to convey the temporal implications of predictive genetic testing for kin beyond the time of taking the test and getting the result. Due to limited space, this longitudinal focus has precluded the examination of all research participants who took part in the study. Use of the present tense, as in the expression 'currently untested', refers to the time of interviewing. Names underlined connote family members who took part actively in the research as interviewees.

Families whose experiences are described in this book include:

THE JEFFRYS FAMILY (Chapter 3)
Dylan, mid 40s, senior manager, has tested negative after his mother, Shirley, has been diagnosed with HD. Dylan is married to Ruth. They parent two adolescent children, Michael and Sandy. Scotland.

THE MCDONALD FAMILY (Chapter 3)
Sam, 50 years, retired schoolteacher. Has tested positive (paternal transmission), currently pre-symptomatic, divorcee and single mother to daughter Belinda ('at risk', currently untested). West Yorkshire.

THE WILLIAMS FAMILY (Chapter 3, 5)
Lucy, 56 years, works in fashion and beauty business. Has tested positive (paternal transmission), currently early symptomatic, married to Rupert, and mother of Laurie, 24, tested positive and Hanno, 22, tested negative. Cornwall.

THE OPIE FAMILY (Chapter 4, 6)
Daisy, 26 years, homemaker. Has tested positive (maternal transmission through Mary), lives with boyfriend Greg Duggan, a self-employed taxi-driver. The couple parent three 'at risk' children, all aged under 7 years (Jamie, Rosa, Penny). Daisy's sister, Liz, remains untested. Southampton.

THE DALEY FAMILY (Chapter 4, 6)
Isobel, 38 years, ex-receptionist. Currently full-time carer to her symptomatic husband, Bruno (early 40s, ex-business executive) whose father Oliver, divorcee of Bruno's

mother, <u>Susie</u>, lives alone coping with his advancing HD symptoms. Isobel and Bruno have two young 'at risk' children, Stefan and Louise. Stefan has Down's syndrome. Dorset.

THE KINGSTON/RICHARDSON FAMILY (Chapter 5)

<u>Mabel Richardson</u> (civil servant) <u>Nelly Richardson</u> (mother to two pre-school children) are sisters, 22 and 21 respectively. Both have tested negative. Their mother <u>Elene</u>, 40 years, is symptomatic (maternal transmission through her late mother Ann, married to Charles) and one of six siblings (née <u>Kingston</u>), five of whom have been diagnosed with HD (<u>Pam</u>, <u>Ted</u>, Elene are in the early stages of illness; their two brothers have committed suicide). Elene and Pam are the genetic parents of eleven offspring between them, all of whom, besides Mabel and Nelly, are 'at risk' children (i.e. their genetic status regarding predisposition to HD is currently unknown). <u>Rex</u> (self-employed market trader), who is married to <u>Claire</u> is the only Kingston sibling not to have inherited HD. Rex has five children (by implication unaffected by HD) by his ex-wife, but whom he parents with Claire. Rex and Claire currently have one child that is their genetic mix (also by implication unaffected by HD). North Yorkshire.

Notes

1 Thinking futures

1. Obituary of Elizabeth Gille, 'The book of the living', *The Guardian*, October 15, 1996, p. 15.
2. One UK company, Sciona Ltd, has already attempted to sell genetic tests directly to the British public through eleven Body Shop stores. The tests (for dietary advice tailored to an individual's genetic make up) were withdrawn from sale in May 2002 after numerous scientists denounced them as meaningless and unethical. Following a campaign by GeneWatch UK and the Consumers' Association, most high street retailers stated that they would not sell the tests, though Sciona is still trying to market them via alternative healthcare outlets, nutritionists, complementary practitioners and others (GeneWatch UK 2002a).
3. The vision was published in *Nature* (2003) volume 422. My thanks to Nick McCooke, Chief Executive Officer of Solexa Ltd, a spin out from the University of Cambridge, for pointing out (pers. comm) the extent to which the 'thousand dollar genome' ideal has caught on as a useful hook within biotech companies. Some companies make the prediction that personalised DNA testing may be realised circa 2010.
4. Issues highlighted by the recent campaign work of biotechnology activists and non-governmental organisations (GeneWatch UK 2003; European Group on Ethics in Science and New Technologies 2003; see also Draper 1991).
5. In contrast to carrier testing and susceptibility testing. While carrier testing is used to detect individuals who possess a single copy of a gene following a recessive pattern of inheritance (e.g. cystic fibrosis, sickle conditions or thalassaemia), susceptibility testing is a diluted form of predictive testing whereby certain gene variants indicative of common diseases (such as Alzheimer's disease and diabetes) may be targeted with drug treatments. These classificatory differences are outlined further in the UK Human Genetics Commission (2000).
6. There are many cultural critiques of the routinisation or 'normalisation' of the new biomedical technologies. For recent overview, see Rapp's (1999) analysis of maternal experience and amniocentesis. Routinisation of genetic testing seems inevitable at least initially in Western Europe and the US, with those less developed countries rich enough to implement a biotechnological 'modernisation' programme as the guise of specific health rationales, never that far behind. The availability of sex-selection programmes in parts of India, for example, shows how female

infanticide as gender discrimination can be 'normalised' as a form of economic rationalisation.

7. See, for example, Park 1963; Beattie 1967; Lienhardt 1969; Middleton 1971; Turner 1975; Jules-Rosette 1978; Werbner 1989. The anthropological study of divination, though largely sidelined in the 1960s by monographs on witchcraft and religion, and despite receiving little sustained attention since structuralist-inspired accounts, has nonetheless roused scholarly interest for the great variety of divinatory forms witnessed both within and across cultures. The extent of the variation is already apparent simply from a reading of these classic African materials.

8. On 'therapeutic' divination, early ethnography already conflates divination with diagnosis, equating the figure of the diviner with the skill of the diagnostician. William Morgan (1931) argues that the use of the Western technical term diagnostician for medical diviners implies Navaho medicine is more than simply another ethnographic rendition of 'primitive' medicine. I simply note this as an observation rather than deal in detail with the implications of the bias.

9. This performative/revelatory quality of the oracle is in contrast to omens that need only simple observation, usually of some natural phenomena, and may be further compared with what Western scientists would liken to the given order of 'discovery' versus [the ingenuity of] 'invention'.

10. Note that Nancy Wexler (1989), whose work I mention below, was one of the earliest social science commentators to forge a connection between genetics and prophecy, specifically in the context of medico-scientific research relating to Huntington's Disease. Wexler develops the connection from a cognitive and psychological perspective, but does not go on to develop this conceptually as a specifically cultural critique. Margaret Lock (1998) takes up the conceptual bait from an anthropological stance, but note that where Lock runs omens and oracles together, Evans-Pritchard (1937) took pains to distinguish between the efficacy of each.

11. On the geneticisation of risk, see also critiques by Parsons and Atkinson 1992; Rabinow 1999; Finkler 2003.

12. The technical term penetrance refers to the frequency with which a dominant allele is expressed in the phenotype of the individual carrying it.

13. See in particular Nader's (1996) pioneering critique.

14. In medical and psychological anthropology, narrative ethics has been closely associated with a 'meaning-centred' interpretive approach in which healers, patients and their kin construct and negotiate the meanings of illness or therapy (Brody 1987; Nelson 1997; Mattingly 1998). One of the strengths of this approach, particularly evident in stories about chronic pain and the protracted process of arriving at diagnosis, is the awareness of shifting modalities of time and temporal shapes. 'Little therapeutic plots' based on the rehabilitative techniques of occupational therapists employed in North American institutional settings in the 1970s and 1980s, show for instance how narrative, as the enactment of a constellation of emotions such as hope, fear and desire, defies any simple diachronic structure of movement (Mattingly 1998). In other words, time takes on narrative depth as an anti-linear, anti-sequential trajectory interweaving a remembered past with an anticipated future. Contrary to the grand narrative of the epic or universal 'mytheme', it is the experiences of feeling and embodied *agents* that bring these situated narratives to life.

15. The standardisation of medical pedigrees required not simply the extension of Mendelian theories and tools into human diseases but also the gathering of family trees, which had already started in clinics in the late nineteenth century. Paying special attention to the use of medical records for Huntington's in North America and Japan, Nukaga (2002) analyses how medical practitioners' responses to the diverging interpretations of hereditary diseases led to the standardisation of family information in clinical practices.

16. For details outlining the transnational collaborative science efforts that led to the discovery of the HD marker and localisation of the gene, see Wexler (1996).

17. For clinical details of HD, see further Harper (1996). For a general historiography of the disease and epidemiological incidence, see Hayden (1981). Besides Huntington's there are at present only a few 'single gene' diseases for which predictive (pre-symptomatic) genetic testing is feasible such as inherited breast and ovarian cancer (BRCA1 and BRCA2), familial adenomatous polyposis, cystic fibrosis. Prenatal testing is possible currently for Tay-Sachs, Gaucher's disease, sickle-cell disease, HD, phenylketonuria, neurofibromatosis, Fragile X, early onset Alzheimer's disease.

18. For further details on method, see Appendix.

19. Other personal accounts and biographical materials relating to HD are explored in Klein 1982; Gray 1995; Leal-Pock 1998. A number of experimental dramatic works and fictional pieces have also explored certain aspects of HD lived experience. See for instance Kyle 1985; Vine 1989; Sawyer 1998; Rubalcaba 1996.

20. See, for example, Chadwick 1993; Marteau and Richards 1996; Wiggins *et al.* 1992; Bundey 1997.

21. See, for example, Richards 1997; Davison 1997.

2   Approaching translocations

1. The terms of the 1997 Declaration (UNESCO 1997a), formally adopted by the General Conference at its twenty-ninth session on 11 November 1997, were agreed after several drafts and meetings of the in-house International Bioethics Committee whose expert witnesses and consultations spanned several years (1994–1997). A Legal Commission and various medical and non-medical consultative experts, predominantly lawyers and philosophers, supplemented the work of the IBC. The final adoption of the draft version had been observed additionally by several intergovernmental and international NGOs (e.g. the Council of Europe, the Council for International Organisations of Medical Sciences [CIOMS] and the World Federation of Scientific Workers [WFSW]).

2. See paragraph 2 of 'Explanatory Note' of Annex 1(B) of UNESCO (1997b).

3. The proliferation of new ethics codes since the inception of the Nuremberg Code in 1947 (reflected in UN Declarations, Council of Europe Conventions, the European Charter, EU Directives, national protocol, guidelines and non-statutory recommendations) and the attendant professionalisation of the 'expert' bioethicist serving professional standard setting bodies (e.g. institutional review boards) provides another site for the 'familiarising' or 'domesticating' work of cultural translation (Fox 2000:5). Codification makes cultural continuity explicit as another agenda of democratic legitimacy: if it is said that patient rights are protected, the explosion of the medical ethos simultaneously could be said to 'save' the face of moral philosophy (see Tröhler and Reiter-Theil 1998). 'Harmonisation' serves its own ends in the national domain, as well as across the international stage.

4. Canada was the only dissenting Member State to withdraw from the proceedings claiming there had been insufficient time during the meeting for extensive international debate of the various articles. Particular concern was expressed about the Declaration's omission of newly emerging procedures such as future possibilities for human cloning and germ-line intervention. See Annex 2 of UNESCO (1997b).

5. The Drafting Committee, as sub-committee of the Committee of Governmental Experts, charged itself with the work of drawing together ('reconciling') and summarising the various opinions of the state representatives. The meetings were closed to uninvited observers.

6. In the manner of Visweswaran (1994:213) and Clifford (1997), for example. I would like to acknowledge Lila Abu-Lughod for assisting the project of 'halfie' self-fashioning (Abu-Lughod 1991), if only to convince of the impossibility of ever realising a neat division between ethnographic identities shaped in the immediacy of the field and beyond.

7. I borrow the term 'truth squads' from Dorothy Nelkin's (1996:98) critique.

8. For specific examples of alignments between different science camps, see Segerstrale's discussion (2001) of objectivist Enlightenment and value-informed hyper-Enlightenment science approaches.

9. This is a broad 'brush stroke' account of general trends and I apologise to colleagues in philosophy and related fields for drawing what some inevitably will see as an over-synthesised précis.

10. However, there is a major proviso to be added. The argument that cultural relativism has avoided a sustained body of genuinely comparative analysis is a separate issue. Likewise it is misleading to run together particularism and a propensity against evaluative judgement as *necessarily* linked effects of the morality that is cultural relativism.

11. See, in particular, Scheper-Hughes (1995) reply to D'Andrade (1995) as part of the opposing positions adopted in the moral 'objectivity and militancy' debate.

12. On the genesis of bioethics and its fundamental grounding in Western law and philosophy, see commentary by Jonsen (1991) and Rothman (1991). Fox (1990) details specifically the 'American-ness' of bioethics and the field's deep-rooted assumptions in concepts of individualism.

13. However, the increased attention in recent years of medical anthropology to Western biomedicine has in certain cases been marked by a heightened concern with ethical questions, as detailed by Hahn and Gaines 1985; Lock and Gordon 1988; Mol and Berg 1998.

14. For classic statement see Beauchamp and Childress (1979). Also Gillon (1994).

15. Spin-offs include Lewontin, Rose and Kamin (1984) and Kitcher (1985). A comprehensive review of the respective ideological positions of the controversy is detailed in Segerstråle (2001); meanwhile Rabinow's (1996) anthropological critique identifies the epistemic shift from sociobiology to biosociality.

16. As an aside, 'the proper study of mankind' happens also to be the title of a retrospective anthology of essays written by the Oxford philosopher Isaiah Berlin, (edited by Henry Hardy and Roger Hausheer [Pimlico edition, 1998]). Hausheer's 'Introduction' of Berlin's contribution to cultural history, political theory and to the possibilities for a 'science of man' (1998:xxv) passes by an anthropological link even as it celebrates Berlin's life-long fascination with human problems, especially questions of human identity and value. 'Few modern thinkers have been as aware as Berlin of *the central categories that constitute our notion of human beings*' (1998:xxvii, emphasis added).

17. For humans the entire code, or the complete book of life, is believed to be some 3,000 million letters long and is said to constitute what geneticists call the 'full text'. Kay's (1999) historical overview of representations of 'the book of life' and the project of 'writing' nature traces antecedents to classical antiquity. For contrasting positions see Watson 1980; Olby 1974; Sinsheimer 1967; see also Keller (1992) on the rhetorical power of 'secrets of life' and anthropological counterpoint in Konrad (2003a).

18. See for example Fox Keller 1995; Doyle 1997; Knorr-Cetina 1999; Kay 2000.

19. Besides genetics, the information metaphor was imported into other biological and non-biological fields, for instance the development of communication theory in immunology and the experimentation of cybernetic models in endocrinology. Outside of biology, Roman Jakobson and others made attempts to recast structural linguistics as a science based on information theory.

20. As Rose (1999:188) notes: 'it is likely to be on the terrain of ethics that our most important political disputes will have to be fought for the foreseeable future'.

21. Today the science of comparative genomics also means that the *proper* study of mankind (after Edmund Leach) is transmuted into a theoretical critique of anthropocentrism and the manifold interdependencies between human and non-human life forms. Study of these particular interdependencies is beyond the focus of this book.

22. See for example Strathern 1992a and 1992b; Franklin 1997, Franklin and Ragoné 1998; Edwards *et al.* 1999, Edwards 2000; Rapp 1991, 1995, 1997, 1999; Becker 2000; Konrad 2003a and b, 2005).

23. See, for example, Barth 1975; Harris 1978; Rosaldo 1980; James 1988; Overing and Passes 2000.

24. For example Strathern 1968; Brodwin 1996; Das 1994; Lock 1995; Farmer 1999. One sees how the wide-ranging regional disparity of these references speak directly to Firth's point, mentioned earlier, that the anthropological study of value has been unsystematic as a conceptual programme of dedicated research. See examples in Howell (1997) as preliminary corrective.

25. On the suggestiveness and limitations of the mapping metaphor see Lippman 1992; Balmer 1996; Rothman 1998.

26. See http://genome.cse.ucsc.edu/

27. The following account is based on conversations with and observations of British molecular biologists and geneticists working in both research and clinical capacities, mainly university departments and teaching hospitals. I have drawn additionally from various genetic textbooks and manuals such as Sudbery 1998; Mange and Mange 1999; Hodson 1994.

28. In family genetics, 'linkage' refers to the coinheritance of genetic markers (such as DNA polymorphisms) with the disease phenotype in those families with multiple affected members. Consistent coinheritance of the marker with the disease in many families indicates that it is in close proximity to the actual disease gene, and as such is said to be 'linked'.

29. *Chiasma* refers to the point at which half of a duplicated chromosome (or chromatid) joins another chromatid during cross-over. When a chromatid belonging to one chromosome remains attached at one or more points to a chromatid from the other, this gives the appearance of a cross; hence the chromosome bridges are called *chiasmata*.

30. Metaphase 1 and 2 and anaphase 1 and 2 correspond to the twofold division of the cell during meiosis: whereas the cell divides twice, the chromosomes divide only once. The spindle itself is a structure of minute fibres that appears in the cell's

nucleus and is said to be 'involved in organising the movement of chromosomes during cell division' (Hodson 1994).

31. The term 'jumping gene' refers to genes that move *within* chromosomes. See note 30.

32. Additionally, the rhetoric of transposition, metabolic pathways, transduction, and even the message-encoding metaphor of transcription itself all convey the possibilities of location and movement. Transposition refers to the movement of a transposon or other movable sequence of deoxyribonucleic acid (DNA) from one place in the genome to another. (Transposons are mobile DNA sequences similar to a 'jumping gene'. Transposons, however, unlike jumping genes, leave a copy of their *original* position when they move to a new site. Barbara McClintock should be credited with this early destabilisation of the gene, as first perceived in her work on the genetics of maize. See Evelyn Fox Keller's [1983] biography.) The operator region or so-called 'operon' embraces the idea of metabolic pathways, and transduction refers to the transfer of genetic information from one bacterium to another when carried by a bacteriophage. Transcription, the first phase of protein synthesis whereby DNA is converted into ribonucleic acid (RNA), is said to commence in the area known as the *promoter region* or 'at the start codon a few bases *further downstream*' (Hodson 1994:255).

33. In somatic cells, translocations effect duplication (as partial trisonomy) or deletion (as partial monosomy).

34. This may lead to a chromosome imbalance, for example a minority of Down's syndrome cases result from an unbalanced translocation caused by trisomy (additional copy) for part of chromosome 21.

35. This follows in spirit the work of certain American critical theorists on the role of metaphor in science and the use of scientific metaphors for the modelling of cultural critique. Doyle (1997) and Haraway (2000) for instance detail in extensive fashion how the discourses of molecular biology often 'slip up' as unthought gaps in knowledge production. By extending certain metaphors in scientific discourse to broader social and institutional fields of power, Keller (1995), Kay (2000) and Traweek (1992) all discuss versions of 'trafficking across borders' between genetics and embryology, physics and biology, biology and the cyber-sciences (cf. also Goodman *et al.* 2003).

36. From a different angle I thus take up Arjun Appadurai's point about the production of ethnographies that seek to emphasise a diversity of themes capable of being fruitfully pursued in any place and for which the 'essence' of a particular place 'reflect[s] the temporary *localisation* of ideas from *many* places' (Appadurai 1992:44 emphasis original). In refusing to see the power of representational essentialisms as strategies of 'metonymic freezing', Appadurai cuts into the conventional place/image nexus, and other similar rhetorical tropes for inter-cultural comparison. The view that 'India' can be 'placed' and summoned up in the anthropological imagination as though it were simply isomorphic with 'hierarchy' for instance, or the essentialising strategy that connects 'Melanesia' necessarily to exchange forms are dead Eurocentric fantasies that operate as conceptual impositions.

3 Foretelling foreknowledge

1. In the following accounts all names of research participants (referred to alternately as interlocutors, testees, counselees, 'at risk' persons, [in-marrying] partners,

carers) are pseudonyms. To protect adult informants and children's identities, I have felt it necessary to change, in certain places, only *minor* biographical details within any given family. Since I have made every effort to stay as close as possible to the verbatim record, none of these author-imposed changes distort the drift of interlocutors' own reported experiences. Nor do they affect my core argument. Unless otherwise stated, the ethnographic present refers to the time of my interviewing.

2. The up-beat optimism of Sam's doctor may be attributed to the particular timing of her test result in 1993. It is whilst Sam is waiting for her result that news of the 'isolation' of the HD gene (as the identification of an expanded CAG repeat) is announced by the international medico-scientific community.

3. These numbers refer to the extensiveness of the trinucleotide CAG expansion repeats characterising the HD gene. Especially significant since, in the case of Huntington's, the so-called 'grey area' of CAG repeats may set up a narrow margin of error or uncertainty in the medical transmission (i.e. false positives and false negatives) of predictive results. Given that in a small number of cases an intermediate allele within the range of 36–41 repeats represents an inconclusive result, individuals whose numbers fall within this range may or may not develop HD in the future (see Brinkman *et al.* 1997). Laurie's number is at the upper end of the uncertainty cusp and he has been told his positive prognosis contains no margin of uncertainty.

4. Religion does, however, feature heavily on the (largely US) discussion lists like Hunt Diss. Compare also to the more generalised statements on the links between religious influence and genetic decision-making or the use of genetic information that can be glossed from large survey studies such as the People's Panel conducted by MORI Social Research (Human Genetics Commission 2001). Note though that public responses to hypothetical surveys generally indicate attitudes, not behaviour.

5. Philosopher Karl Popper viewed the history of Western science as a sequence of conjectures, refutations, revised conjectures and additional refutations, and argued that empirical method depends upon exposing a theory to the possibility of being falsified. On the liabilities of veracity and truth manipulations as a version of kinship ethics, see, however, Chapter 4.

6. A note on sources. The expression 'ritual as experimental technology' is elaborated by Whyte (1997:205–8) as part of a theoretical agenda on the 'pragmatics of misfortune' originally applied to HIV/AIDS discourses amongst the Nyole of Uganda. Whyte herself acknowledges the explicitly political dimensions of ritual outlined by Jean and John Comaroff (1993) in relation to their fieldwork engagement with changing political conditions in post-colonial South Africa. By referring to ritual as 'an experimental technology intended to affect the flow of power in the universe' (J. and J. Comaroff 1993:xxx), ritual action is aligned here conceptually with specifically cultural responses to social transformation. Building on Whyte's deployment of the Comaroffs' notion of transformative 'experimental technology', I further appropriate the expression from the Africanists to explore the specific workings of prophetic genetics as a form of ritual in technoscientific predictive medicine. Compare with DeHart's analysis (1997) that arrives at problems of ritual through the philosophy of technology.

7. The procedures of genetic counselling and the testing protocol are summarised in the official HD Guidelines. *Guidelines for the Molecular Genetics Predictive Test in HD* was originally drawn up by a committee consisting of representatives of the International Huntington Association (IHA) and the World Federation of Neurology (WFN) Research Group on Huntington's Chorea in 1985. They were subsequently

revised after the successful location of the gene by scientists in 1993 and published in the *Journal of Medical Genetics* 1994 (31):555–59.)

The ideals of value-neutrality and non-directiveness inform the dominant approaches to genetic counselling. Based on client-centred focus, these twin ideals are rooted in professional self-distancing from eugenic practices of population 'improvement', and supposedly enacted through a non-judgemental and supportive relationship between the counsellor and counselee. The difficulty, if not impossibility, of implementing these ideals in actual practice, however, is acknowledged both from within certain quarters of the genetics counselling profession (e.g. Clarke 1991, 1997, Michie and Marteau 1996), as well as by critical commentators from the social sciences (e.g. Chadwick 1993; Rapp 1989, 1999; Petersen and Bunton 2002).

In terms of genetic policy formulation, the tension between non-directive counselling ideals and practice has been noted (e.g. the Nuffield Council on Bioethics [1998:80]), although to date there has been no substantive Consultation process inviting public response nor any critical review examining changes within the genetics counselling profession. In the light of the increased availability and use of genetic tests for adults, children, potential parents and possibly even potential marriage partners, these tensions look set to become increasingly prominent as ethico-political matters that propel science into the public space of the 'agora' (Nowotny *et al.* 2002). Since the marshalling, collection, control and dissemination of information by genetic counsellors constitutes another kind of genetic 'technology', to be able to engage with and reflect upon how such information is deployed, manipulated and framed as cultural value opens a dynamic relationship for the contextualisation of knowledge as 'socially robust'.

8. Acronyms are a common device of this language framework effecting distancing of professionals as knowledgeable 'experts' (an implied if not enacted separation between counsellor and counselee). Rapp was to hear the following admission by one workshop leader at a counselling conference: 'We all speak in anagrams [acronyms]. Can you remember when you learned to talk about LMP, AMA, TOP, FISH, PCRs, RFLPs? And when you learned to stop talking about RFLPs [a gene-splicing technology that quickly became obsolete]?' Rapp (1999:62).

9. One may take the associated report on human genetics by The House of Commons Science and Technology Committee (1995) as evidence of the discursive subtlety with which these tensions are perceived and played out in much clinical practice. Whilst acknowledging the transformative effects attached to the oracular power of genetic testing technologies, at the same time the report underscores this same fundamental contradiction of illusory expectation: the apparent ubiquity of the information-seeking individual as autonomous subject. Paragraph 79 (1995:xxxviii) cautions that 'it is important that such [genetic] information is given only when *the person concerned is certain that they wish to receive it*' (emphasis added).

10. In its submission to the Human Genetics Commission Consultation on genetic tests supplied direct to the public, GIG (The Genetic Interest Group) noted similarly. 'Individuals should not be compelled to take part in such discussions; there are some well-informed individuals who may wish to avail themselves of a DNA test and nothing more, and they should be allowed to do so' (see HGC 2003:31).

11. The current vision of 'spreading learning opportunities' is encapsulated by the proposal to establish an NHS Genetics Education and Development Centre affiliated to the NHSU, the university for the NHS. The Development Centre is framed as at once a cohesive entity capable of extending beyond itself; its

objective being to 'act as a catalyst and help drive and co-ordinate activity' at the same time as it seeks to link up to 'all those bodies and organisations responsible for determining learning needs' (Department of Health 2003:49–50).

12. On the one hand, the attending physician could achieve moral absolution for himself in cases of a patient's sudden death. Simply by claiming to have 'foreseen' an impending loss of life, the physician could escape blame for medicine's (and indeed his own) apparent failure (Edelstein 1967:66–67, 75). Prognosis was in this sense a convenient professional get-out, a manoeuvring away from sworn codes of accountability and the silent 'confession' of having insufficient knowledge about knowledge (usually disease aetiology). And yet, it was this very ability of Hippocratic physicians to summon knowledge as prognosis (even, apparently, without the need to ask the patient specific personal questions) that counted as evidence of professional skill itself. Those who could establish a medical history and advance a prognosis were looked upon favourably as gifted healers, in contrast to the inferiority accorded to common quacks and unreliable diviners. Prognosis was, then, a revered emblem of Greek social prestige, a way for professional fame to be carried across space and time as the 'person' of the itinerant physician moved from household to household. As the trust of confidence others relayed to him fed his 'reputation', so the person of the physician came to be linked intimately with this special ability to prognosticate (see Lloyd 1978:170).

13. Experiencing a sense of bereavement in anticipation of one's own death informs some of the ethnographic literature on AIDS activism, palliative care, 'right-to-die' initiatives and the drawing up of 'advanced directives', as well as patients' narratives of dealing with chronic illness more generally (e.g. Kleinman 1988; Jackson 2000).

14. Note that doctors are much more likely to proffer prognosis when the patient *expressly* asks for this. See Christakis (1999:106) and Monks's (2000) analysis of the 'phatic' quality of chatty talk between doctors and patients.

15. The potential for a productive collision between theory making and confession derives more broadly from the contributions of feminist epistemology to the conceptualisation of narrative theory (see Skultans 2000). For example, expanding the tradition of 'empathic witnessing' (Kleinman 1988:154), Geyla Frank's (2000) cultural biography of disability is refreshingly honest in its reflections on ethnographic anxiety and narrative ambiguity in the research process. Likewise, Katharine Young's narrativised camouflaging of the (otherwise sequestered) self temporarily transforms the (critical gaze) of the researcher into 'a species of disembodiment' during patients' gynaecological examinations (Young 1997:4). Outside of biomedicine, methodological and theoretical considerations feature strongly in the accounts of critical reflexivity informing the auto/biographical commentaries in Okely and Callaway (1992) and Reed-Danahy (1997).

16. On narratives as a moral device for allocating blame see Mattingly (1998:4–5) and Lewis (2000).

17. Theorised *inter alia* by Zola 1972; Illich 1977; Taussig 1980; Frankenberg 1980; Scheper-Hughes and Lock 1990; Good 1994.

4 Tracing genealogies of non-disclosure

1. Beyond the fixed protocol of genetic counselling, clinicians do not discuss in any considerable detail the kinds of burdens set up by these disclosure 'duties' nor do they tend to draw explicitly upon the emotional experiences of past testees (cf Green *et al.* 1997; Kessler 1979; Bartels *et al.* 1993). Outside the field of medical

genetics, however, various ethnographic evidence on illness experience already points to the considerable difficulties persons may experience in disclosing intimate medical knowledge amongst close kin. Rare insights are provided for instance by Slomka (1992) on the pluralistic 'bargaining' of end-of-life interventions and the ensuing 'cascade' of kinship decisions. Compare with Frank *et al.* (1998) on decision-making amongst elderly Korean Americans; Marshall *et al.* (1991) on HIV disclosure and Gordon's work (1990, 1994) on cancer communication within Italian families. On the broader discursive significance of kinship duties, see by way of analogy Lori Andrews' (1997) work on contemporary adoption procedures in the US. Andrews argues that because genetic diseases are not contagious and therefore cannot implicate a particular agent as causative social entity, an individual with a genetic mutation is under no legal obligation to warn relatives. The patient cannot be said to be *causing* a potential risk to relatives since affected kin (i.e. non-affines) will be predisposed to inherit the gene irrespective of what the patient him or herself does (Andrews 1997; cf. Pelias 1991). Such social science commentary helps to take the debate in a different direction: immediately, it highlights the important point that responsibilities to other relatives cannot simply be owed on the basis of a biological bond *per se.*

2. Unambiguous circumstances involve 'exceptions'. Disclosure to a third party may be required by statute, in the public interest, or in connection with judicial proceedings.

3. As the Human Genetics Commission observes in its Discussion Document on personal genetic information: 'Such breaches would only be made if the person in possession of the information had tried unsuccessfully to persuade the patient to agree to its disclosure and if, *on balance*, the harm caused by non-disclosure is thought to outweigh the harm caused to the patient by breaching confidentiality' (Human Genetics Commission 2000:17, emphasis added). The opposing view would express caution and care over 'the breaking of confidentiality in contexts where professionals are much keener to provide services than many family members are to use them' (Nuffield Council on Bioethics 1998:51).

4. The very problematisation of the disclosure of personal medical and genetic information closely supports the Western-derived medico-ethical *doxa* of respect for the person and the associated principle of individual autonomy. In turn these values are based on highly particularistic conceptions of personhood as self-unitary and self-determining (for mainstream views see Beauchamp and Childress 1994; Fox 1990; Kuczewski and Polansky 2000).

5. Chadwick (1997) does introduce the concept of solidarity into the discussion, noting it too informs the right to know/right not to know debates. The important point however is that the theorisation of claims to solidarity as forms of communitarianism or mutuality has been overshadowed by the emphasis attached to rights to confidentiality and privacy, as though these rights must be invested exclusively in the privileged entity known as the 'individual'.

6. Acts of disclosure comprise much more of a symbiotic and interdependent relationship than medics commonly acknowledge. Clinical and research staff *need* to extract certain individual life history and family information through the medical genealogies they collect, for example. There is a point of methodological concern here. Because information is communicated between practitioners and patients under the cover of confidentiality in Western health contexts, it is extremely difficult for 'outsiders' in their research capacity as detached observers to access and gather critical information about these restricted sites. Research by non-medics documenting the nature of the transmission and reception of sensitive personal information is therefore practically non-existent. The transcripts of Young (1997)

detailing hospital-based praxis for gynaecological examination and surgery are notable in this regard.

7. The term 'negotiated relevance' has been applied fruitfully to the production of local knowledge for decision-making in international public health contexts. See Yoder (1997).

8. 'What is truth? A mobile army of metaphors, metonyms, anthropomorphisms . . . Truths are illusions about which it has been forgotten that they are illusions, worn-out metaphors . . .' (Nietzsche 1873:250).

9. Except insofar as these practices are defined negatively, namely as the failure to offer or promote one particular medicine (e.g. hospital medicine) over another (e.g. Islamic medicine).

10. McCallum's argument, more broadly, addresses the question of the integrated totality of the body that acts as 'mind'; in other words according to Cashinahua folk understanding, mind is a diffuse corporeal experience. Contra to the Western attribution of intelligence to the neuro-chemical structure that is the human brain, the Cashinahua appear not to think in terms of a discrete physical entity that can be located in a particular region of the body or body part.

11. Corresponding to care-based approaches informing feminist (bio)ethics that question likewise the relevance of adherence to fixed ethical principles (e.g. Noddings 1984).

12. See Genetic Interest Group (1998:16).

5 Reproducing exclusion

1. This implication of kin in the time of others' anticipatory illness bears upon the earlier discussion in Chapter 3 on the false dichotomy of 'pre-symptomatic' versus 'symptomatic' classifications.

2. See, for example, 'Fury at plan to sell off DNA secrets', *The Observer*, 23 September 2001, p. 1.

3. 'The eclecticism we find in Wana magic and shamanship derives from an emphasis on innovation and entrepreneurship in dealings with hidden dimensions of reality' (Atkinson 1989:65).

4. See especially Desjerlais (1992) on Nepali shamans and Jakobsen (1999) on new shamanic movements in Greenland.

5. 'The items being returned to and removed from the patients' bodies in these texts belong to a dimension of reality that lies beyond most people's perception but at the same time concerns their very survival' (Atkinson 1989:90). One could say this aesthetic of therapeutic translocation captures something of the spirit of experimental gene therapy. Like shamanistic endeavour, genetic therapy is a modality that circumvents interiorised versus exteriorised dichotomies through the movement and replacement of certain bodily parts (though here mediation would be performed not just by medics but by the [technicised] interventionary properties of certain virus vectors).

6 Relinquishing exclusion

1. In the UK, the treatment is currently available at a limited number of specialist-licensed clinics and accessible only to those couples with the pre-knowledge one reproductive partner may transmit a so-called 'serious' genetic

condition. Of interest is the way such knowledge concedes altered reproductive agency. Note that members of the UK Human Genetics Commission endorsed their Consultation Paper's inclination to leave undefined what exactly can be termed as 'serious enough for inclusion' in a PGD protocol list (Human Fertilisation and Embryology Authority/Advisory Committee on Genetic Testing 1999:9; Human Genetics Commission 2001a:2–3). Currently biopsied cells from the testee can be tested for about two dozen genetically determined diseases. Specifically, only those IVF-cultured embryos that have been found not to carry the affected gene after fertilisation, cell biopsy and diagnosis are transferred to the prospective mother. For overviews of PGD techniques and key developments, see the summary and comprehensive bibliography in Harper and Delhanty (2000) representing data prepared for the European Society for Human Reproduction and Embryology PGD Consortium Steering Committee (1999).

At the time of writing the HFEA (2003) has issued a recommendation to restrict sex selection procedures to medical grounds alone. However, the possible deployment of the technique in the future for non-medical reasons (e.g., selection, besides such sex-linked diseases as Duchenne's muscular dystrophy, for 'gender preference' or the selective enhancement of certain 'desirable' traits) continues to create dissensus amongst many parties. Difference of view amongst 'the prospective public' is to be heard from certain parents-to-be, healthcare professionals, scientists, religious and legal commentators, activist campaign groups, many of whom may have parallel identities as citizen, parent and professional.

2. On assembling the figure of the embryo through the persistence of its cultural elision, see Franklin (1997) and Becker (2000).
3. Exclusion PGD testing entails the genetic cross-comparison of the grandparental allele with that of the embryo whereas prenatal exclusion testing deploys linked DNA probes. See further Bloch and Hayden 1987; Sermon *et al.* 1998 for clinical exposition.
4. Prenatal exclusion testing adds further unresolved complexity to an already risky procedure. In cases of autosomal dominant inheritance such as HD, it carries the risk of terminating an unaffected foetus because following a positive test there is as much chance of aborting a normal foetus as an affected one. For this reason, exclusion testing has become more contentious since the HD gene has been identified and has enabled predictive/pre-symptomatic testing.
5. Hence the clinical preference for direct pre-symptomatic testing of the 'at risk' person or PGD exclusion testing which Sermon *et al.* (1998) refer to as 'real' exclusion testing. The latter method determines the absence or presence of a chromosome inherited from the affected grandparent.
6. A number of clinical studies report that when HD at-risk patients undergo prenatal exclusion testing, many women have elected for a late reversal of a previous decision to undergo first-trimester termination. See, for instance, Tolmie *et al.* (1995). Again in this situation, the child's right not to know its genetic heritage may already be compromised before its birth. See Bloch and Hayden 1987; Quarell *et al.* 1987.
7. Such imagery of nested relations derives in part from the anthropological literature on *société à maisons* (house societies) in which houses, as self-contained microcosms, are said to contain both a miniature image of the universe and to set off in turn the whole system of social relations. (The symbolism of the physical house is especially well documented for Southeast Asian and Mesoamerican house societies; see e.g. Lévi-Strauss 1987; Carsten and Hugh-Jones 1995). Such

comparative exercises tell us how the biosocial entity that is the moral person (the 'house', for example) extends well beyond the autonomous, self-bounded conception of the Western-invoked 'embryo' or 'individual'. See, for instance, Gillespie's rendition of the Tzotzil Maya 'nested' house/human body as related microcosmic models 'each individually bounded in its spatial element but simultaneously interpenetrating, one inside another . . . potentially provid[ing] everyone and everything a proper place' (Gillespie 2000:139–40).

8. Rapp (1999:183) offers a similar qualification for her amniocentesis testimonies amongst a diverse group of informants with various religious, ethnic and cultural affiliations (resident in North America).

9. Again I stress that such views are not the understandings of all couples. Some prospective parents, particularly in cases where there is a known risk of HD in either parent, said they would want to go ahead with pre-implantation genetic diagnosis and were arranging to be put on waiting lists for the treatment or trying to raise the necessary finances. Some complained that the service was not more readily available or nationally funded. Here, my point is simply to insist on the need to attend to the many different voices of women and other dissenting subjects. When the form such resistance takes cannot always be articulated clearly in ordinary discourse, then such documentation becomes especially important. As much critical social analysis has shown, forms of resistance agency that appear to confirm the status quo are always much harder to document and conceptualise than the voices of openly articulated dissent.

10. The 'right to disability' has been put forward specifically by congenitally deaf parents who have argued it may be in the long-term interests of their offspring as well as the couple themselves to share the same environmental experiences as their next of kin. See discussion in Silvers (1999) and Connor (2000). Note that in the joint Human Fertilisation and Embryology Authority/Advisory Committee on Genetic Testing Consultation Document on Pre-implantation Genetic Diagnosis' (1999:11), the social reproduction of cultures of disability was recognised as a legitimate possibility. User organisations and activist groups lobbying for disabled people in Germany and the Netherlands have promoted the concept of 'a right to abnormality' on the grounds that diversity sustains and strengthens ideals of community (Hepburn 1998). An important and growing literature is documenting sociological and feminist bioethics rejoinders of genetics in the context of disability rights; see for example, Shakespeare (1998, 1999); Asch (1989, 1993); Silvers (1999).

11. Significantly, I have not been able to establish the date of Oliver's letter, and thus the interval of time between its receipt and its re-activation as source of revelatory knowledge (the formal act of kinship disclosure). Regarding Isobel and Bruno's decision not to disclose news of their forthcoming addition to the family, this is part of a long history of intra-familial disagreement. There have been significant conflicts in the past regarding care arrangements and grandparental assistance, as well as disputes over mobility and how far the couple should reside in terms of geographical distance from their in-laws.

12. On the conventional medical presumption that an unfavourable test result following prenatal diagnosis will lead to an abortion, see Green's (1995) socio-psychological study. Green reports that over one third of a sample of obstetricians said that they generally require a woman to agree to termination of an affected pregnancy before offering prenatal diagnosis.

13. 'Pre-implantation diagnosis for Huntington's Disease', *Huntington's Disease Association Newsletter*, issue 53, p. 13 (1998).

14. As I have been pointing out, Daisy and Isobel's accounts are not isolated incidences. On the very low uptake rates of prenatal diagnosis and abortion for HD generally, see Adam *et al.* 1993; Tolmie *et al.* 1995. For feminist socio-cultural critiques beyond the specifics of HD-related decisions, see Rothman (1986) and Rapp (1999) on non-termination and women's experiences of pregnancy after prenatal diagnosis. See also Nuffield Council of Bioethics (1998:46). Tolmie *et al.* (1995:97) comment that late reversal of a previous decision to undergo first trimester pregnancy termination for a genetic indication is 'uniquely frequent' among couples who have undergone the prenatal exclusion test for HD. The biomedical literature thus recognises that people are resistant in acting upon decisions to *finalise* what is an irreversible (pre-conceptive) exclusion.

15. On pregnancy screening for Down's syndrome and parental choice, see Nuffield Council on Bioethics (1998:50) 'parents should be supported in whatever choice they make'. The view is well meaning but a touch idealistic especially when issues of disability, appraised in terms of the political economy of health rationing, are added into the equation. Not to be forgotten is the 'selectivist' argument that savings resulting from the prevention of 'affected' births would be well recovered by the cost of a genetic screening programme. That it is cheaper to exclude a life than it is to treat a sick person is of course not an unfamiliar ideology, as outlined in Chapter 1.

16. See Nuffield Council on Bioethics (1998:5.32). For a concise overview of the moral and legal debates concerning the genetic testing of children, see Davis (2001:69–87). See also positions expressed by Harper and Clarke (1990) writing in their capacity as clinical geneticists.

17. Isobel's decision happens to be grounded in a particular genealogical chain of potential successive male inheritance. Recent clinical research has found a correlation between inheritance of HD through the paternal line and increasingly earlier age of onset of the disease. This is described clinically as the phenomenon of 'anticipation'. If inheritance has occurred through the paternal line for successive generations, it is very likely a grandson will show symptoms at a considerably earlier age than his grandfather. Isobel's offspring stand as the fourth *known* generation at risk of HD and since Bruno's age of onset (late 30s) was considerably earlier than that of his biological father, she is concerned to know more about the children's predicament in terms of these *temporal* implications. (Note in conjunction the slipperiness of the term 'late-onset' illness here.)

18. Compare with the earlier discussion in Chapter 4 on Cashinuhua ethno-epistemology and the moral constitution of bodily knowledge.

19. Mention should be made of a recently conducted ethnographic study in Britain examining genetic knowledge and pre-implantation genetic diagnosis undertaken by Sarah Franklin and Celia Roberts (Department of Sociology, University of Lancaster, UK). Plans are underway to publish material from this substantial study; Franklin and Roberts have also examined the early stages of stem cell research practices in the UK.

7 Concluding remarks

1. The UK GTN is a subgroup of the Genetics Commissioning Advisory Group which coordinates the NHS network of genetic testing laboratories.

2. In which case predictive medicine would produce the effects of cultural iatrogenesis such that prevailing ailments become the unintended or unwanted outcomes of strategies for better health.

3. And what might you think the lead researcher in charge of this study is reported to have said about such precocity? Nothing unpredictable, of course. Spotting talent early, he remarked, would mean that fewer educational resources need be wasted. 'Not all children can benefit from a university education' (Utley 2003:2). No coincidence the reportage found its way onto the front page of the leading quality weekly newspaper for higher education in the UK.

4. See Coghlan (2000).

5. DNA databanks currently exist in various forms and are subject to different national legislatures or guidelines in Australia, Canada, Estonia, Iceland, Sweden, UK and the USA.

6. UK Biobank, for example, a project co-funded by the Department of Health, the Wellcome Trust and the Medical Research Council, is designed to collect data and blood samples for genetic analysis from 500,000 men and women volunteers aged between 45–69.

7. In practical terms, the objective is to accumulate data on health outcomes. So far as UK Biobank is concerned, information aggregation will be realised as a long-term follow up of the cohort via National Health Service medical records.

8. The Human Genetics Commission (HGC) intends to report its recommendations on genetic profiling at birth to the Department of Health by the end of 2004 after conducting an initial analysis of the issues in conjunction with the National Screening Committee.

9. As part of the National Health Service 'Integrated Care Records Service' (ICRS). Consumer autonomy may be further advanced in the US where federal legislation promotes the genetic testing of all newborns. Thirty-three states carry out programmes that test infants at birth for a number of conditions, including testing for the recessive disorder sickle cell disease (SCD) (Lane 1994).

10. Contrast with the European Convention on Human Rights and Biomedicine [Oviedo Convention, 1997] which enshrines the legal right to know or not to know predictive genetic information based on the principle of informational self-determination. See Chapter 4, Article 12. See further note 14 below.

11. Marketed in the UK by Health Interlink Ltd and available via some alternative health practitioners and GPs, the 'Cardio' profile includes a test for common variations in the ApoE gene (GeneWatch UK 2002b).

12. Although there are laws in the UK that protect the confidentiality of personal information and prevent discrimination against people with existing disabilities, these do not address the complex issues relating to genetic information. (The Human Rights Act [1998] may be relevant in protecting the privacy of genetic information regarding respect for private and family life, however it is not yet clear how British jurisdication would apply the human rights principles in this context.) While there is presently no national legislation in the UK supporting genetic privacy, anti-genetic discrimination legislation applies to Australia (The Genetic Privacy and Non-Discrimination Bill, 1998); Austria (The Gene Technology Act, 1995); Denmark (Act on the Use of Health Information in the Labour Market, 1996); France (Law on Respect for the Human Body, 1994); Netherlands (The Medical Checks Act of 1997 which prohibits the use of pre-symptomatic genetic tests for serious, untreatable conditions); and Norway (The Act Relating to the Application of Biotechnology in Medicine, 1994). A particularly challenging and sensitive area for future regulation concerns the definition of 'disability' and its association (or otherwise) with the emerging classificatory order of the

'pre-symptomatic'. The UK Disability Discrimination Act (1995) extends protection to employees with 'faulty genes' but only if they are currently disabled or have been disabled in the past. It does not cover people who have a susceptibility to ill health in the future. The key cultural issue here for bioethics policy analysis and regulation turns on whether or not it would be appropriate to include people with no presently identifiable symptoms under the definitional rubric of 'disability'.

Bibliography

Abu-Lughod, Lila 1991. 'Writing against culture'. In Richard G. Fox (ed.) *Recapturing Anthropology: Working in the Present*, Sante Fe, NM: School of American Research.

Adam, S., Wiggins, S., Whyte, P., Bloch, M., Shokeir, M., Soltan, H., Meschino, W., Summers, A., Suchowersky, O., and Welch, J. 1993. 'Five year study of pre-natal testing for HD: demand, attitude and pyschological assessment'. *Journal of Medical Genetics* 30: 549–56.

Advisory Committee on Genetic Testing 1997. *Genetic Testing for Late Onset Disorders. Consultation Paper*, London: Department of Health.

Advisory Committee on Genetic Testing 1998. *Report on Genetic Testing for Late Onset Disorders*. London: Department of Health.

Andrews, Lori B. 1997. 'Gen-etiquette: genetic information, family relationships, and adoption'. In Rothstein, M. (ed.) *Genetic Secrets. Protecting Privacy and Confidentiality in the Genetic Era*, pp. 255–80. New Haven, CT: Yale University Press.

Appadurai, Arjun 1992. 'Putting hierarchy in its place'. In G. Marcus (ed.) *Rereading Cultural Anthropology*, London: Duke University Press.

Ardener, Edwin 1989. *The Voice of Prophecy and Other Essays*. Edited by Malcolm Chapman. Oxford: Basil Blackwell.

Armstrong, D. 1995. 'The rise of surveillance medicine'. *The Sociology of Health and Illness* 17: 393–404.

Armstrong, D., Michie, S., and Marteau, T. 1998. 'Revealed identity: a study of the process of genetic counselling'. *Social Science and Medicine* 47, 11: 1653–8.

Asch, Adrienne 1989. 'Reproductive technology and disability'. In Sherrill Cohen and Nadine Taub (eds.) *Reproductive Laws for the 1990s*, pp. 69–125. Clifton, NJ: Humana.

Asch, Adrienne 1993. 'The human genome and disability rights: thoughts for researchers and advocates'. *Disability Studies Quarterly* 13: 3–5.

Asch, Adrienne 1999. 'Prenatal diagnosis and selective abortion: a challenge to practice and policy'. *American Journal of Public Health* 89, 11: 1649–57.

Atkinson, Jane Monnig 1989. *The Art and Politics of Wana Shamanship*, Berkeley, CA: University of California Press.

Bailey, F.G. 1991. *The Prevalence of Deceit*. Ithaca & London: Cornell University Press.

Balmer, Brian 1996. 'The political cartography of the Human Genome Project'. *Perspectives on Science*, 4(3) 98–132.

Bankowski, Z. and A.M. Capron (eds.) 1990. *Genetics, Ethics and Human Values: Human Genome Mapping, Genetic Screening, and Gene Therapy*, Proceedings of the XXIVth CIOMS Conference, Tokyo and Inuyama City, Japan, 22–27 July.

Bartels, Diane M., Bonnie S. Leroy, and Arthur L. Caplan (eds.) 1993. *Prescribing Our Future. Ethical Challenges in Genetic Counselling*. New York: Aldine de Gruyter.

Barth, Fredrik 1975. *Ritual and Knowledge Among the Baktaman of New Guinea*. New Haven, CT: Yale University Press.

Beattie, John 1967. 'Divination in Bunyoro, Uganda'. In John Middleton (ed.) *Magic, Witchcraft and Curing*. Garden City, NY: Natural History Press.

Beauchamp, Tom L. and James F. Childress 1979. *Principles of Biomedical Ethics*. Oxford University Press.

Becker, Gay 2000. *The Elusive Embryo. How Women and Men Approach New Reproductive Technologies*, Berkeley, CA: University of California Press.

Beidelman 1993 [1986]. *Moral Imagination in Kaguru Modes of Thought*, Bloomington, IN: Indiana University Press.

Benatar, S. 1998. 'Imperialism, research ethics and global health', *Journal of Medical Ethics* 24: 221–2.

Bloch, M. and M.R. Hayden 1987. 'Preclinical testing in Huntington's Disease', *American Journal of Medical Genetics* 27: 733–4.

Bok, Sissela 1979. *Lying: Moral Choice in Public and Private Life*, New York: Random House.

Bok, Sissela 1982. *Secrets. On the Ethics of Concealment and Revelation*, New York: Random House.

Bouquet, Mary 1993. *Reclaiming English Kinship: Portuguese Refractions of British Kinship Theory*. Manchester University Press.

Bouquet, Mary 1996. 'Family trees and their affinities: the visual imperative of the genealogical diagram', *Journal of the Royal Anthropological Institute* (N.S.) 2(1): 43–66.

Braude, Peter R., de Vert, G., Evers-Kiebooms, G., Pettigrew, R., and Geraedts, J. 1998. 'Non-disclosure preimplantation genetic diagnosis for Huntington's Disease: practical and ethical dilemmas', *Prenatal Diagnosis* 18: 1422–6.

Brinkman, R., Mezei, M., Theilman, J., Almquist, E., and Hayden, M. 1997. 'The likelihood of being affected by Huntington's Disease by a particular age, for a specific repeat size', *American Journal of Human Genetics* 60: 1202–10.

British Medical Association 1998. *Human Genetics. Choice and Responsibility*. Oxford University Press.

Brody, Howard 1987. *Stories of Sickness*. New Haven, CT: Yale University Press.

Brodwin, Paul 1996. *Medicine and Morality in Haiti*. Cambridge University Press.

Browner, Carole H. 1999. 'On the medicalisation of medical anthropology', *Medical Anthropology Quarterly* 13(2): 134–40.

Browner, Carole H. and Nancy H. Press 1995. 'The normalisation of prenatal diagnostic screening'. In F.D. Ginsburg and R. Rapp (eds.) *Conceiving the New World Order: The Global Politics of Reproduction*, pp. 307–22. Berkeley, CA: University of California Press.

Brunger, F. and A. Lippman 1995. 'Resistance and adherence to the norms of genetic counselling'. *Journal of Genetic Counselling* 4(3): 151–67.

Bundey S. 1997. 'Few psychological consequences of presymptomatic testing for Huntington's Disease', *The Lancet* 349: 4.

Canguilhelm, G. 1966. *Le normal et la pathologique*. Paris: Presses Universitaires de France.

Caplan, P. 2003. *The Ethics of Anthropology*. London: Routledge.

Carsten, J. and S. Hugh-Jones (eds.) 1995. *About the House: Lévi-Strauss and Beyond*. Cambridge University Press.

Chadwick, R. 1993. 'What counts as success in genetic counselling?' *Journal of Medical Ethics* 19: 43–6.

Chadwick, R. 1997. 'The philosophy of the right to know and the right not to know'. In *The Right to Know and the Right Not to Know*. pp. 13–22. Aldershot: Ashgate Publishing Limited.

Chadwick, R. *et al.* 1993. *Ethical Implications of Human Genome Analysis for Clinical Practice in Medical Genetics, With Special Reference to Genetic Counselling*. A Report to the Commission of the European Communities, Cardiff: Centre for Applied Ethics.

Chadwick, R., Levitt, M., and Shickle, D. (eds.) 1997. *The Right to Know and the Right Not to Know*, Aldershot: Ashgate Publishing Limited.

Chadwick, R. and Bock, G. 1990. (eds.) *Human Genetic Information: Science, Law and Ethics*, Chichester: John Wiley & Sons.

Christakis, Nicholas A. 1996. 'The distinction between ethical pluralism and ethical relativism: implications for the conduct of transcultural clinical research'. In Harold Y. Vanderpool (ed.) *The Ethics of Research Involving Human Subjects. Facing the 21st Century*, Frederick, MN: University Publishing Group.

Christakis, Nicholas A. 1999. *Death Foretold: Prophecy and Prognosis in Medical Care*. University of Chicago Press.

Clarke, A. 1991. 'Is non-directive counselling possible?' *The Lancet* 338: 998–1001.

Clarke, A. 1997. 'Outcomes and process in genetic counselling'. In P. Harper and A. Clarke (eds.) *Genetics, Society and Clinical Practice*. Oxford: Bios Scientific Publishers.

Clarke, A. and Parsons, E. (eds.) 1997. *Culture, Kinship and Genes: Towards Cross-Cultural Genetics*. Hampshire: Macmillan Press Ltd.

Clifford, J. 1997. 'Spatial practices: fieldwork, travel, and the disciplining of anthropology'. In A. Gupta and J. Ferguson (eds.) *Anthropological Locations: Boundaries and Grounds of a Field Science*, pp. 185–222. Berkeley, CA: University of California Press.

Coghlan, A. 2000. 'DNA Chips'. *New Scientist*, 11 March.

Comaroff, J. and Comaroff, J. 1993. 'Introduction'. In J. and J. Comaroff (eds.) *Modernity and its Malcontents. Ritual and Power in Postcolonial South Africa*. University of Chicago Press.

Connor, S. 2000. 'Deaf parents seek right to have deaf children', *The Independent*, 21 September, p. 6.

Conrad, Peter and Gabe, J. (eds.) 1999. *Sociological Perspectives on the New Genetics*. Oxford: Blackwell Publishers.

Cox, S.M. and McKellin, W. 1999. ' "There's this thing in our family": predictive testing and the construction of risk for Huntington's Disease'. In P. Conrad and J. Gabe (eds.) *Sociological Perspectives on the New Genetics*, pp. 121–45. Oxford: Blackwell Publishers.

Craufurd, D., Dodge, A., Kerzin-Storrar, L., and Harris, R. 1989. 'Uptake of presymptomatic predictive testing for Huntington's Disease', *Lancet II*: 603–5.

Crossley, M. 1996. 'Choice, conscience, and context'. *Hastings Law Journal* 47(4): 1223–39.

D'Andrade, R. 1995. 'Moral models in anthropology' *Current Anthropology* 36(3): 399–408.

Das, V. 1994. 'Moral orientations to suffering: legitimation, power and healing. Case study victims of the chemical poisoning at Bhopal' In L.C. Chen, A. Kleinman and N. Ware (eds.) *Health and Social Change. An International Perspective*, Cambridge, MA.: Harvard University Press.

Davis, Dena S. 2001. *Genetic Dilemmas. Reproductive Technology, Parental Choices and Children's Futures*, London: Routledge.

Davison, C. 1997. 'Everyday ideas of inheritance and health in Britain: implications for predictive genetic testing'. In A. Clarke and E. Parsons (eds.) *Culture, Kinship and Genes*, pp. 167–74. London: Macmillan Press.

Davison, C., Macintyre, S., and Smith, G.D. 1994. 'The potential social impact of predictive genetic testing for susceptibility to common chromic diseases: a review and proposed research agenda'. *Sociology of Health and Illness* 16(3): 340–71.

DeHart, S. 1997. 'Ritual in technoscientific medicine'. In C. Mitcham (ed.) *Technology and Social Action*, London: JAI, pp. 87–117.

Department of Health 2003. *Our Inheritance, Our Future: Realising the Potential of Genetics in the NHS*. London: DoH.

Desjerlais, R. 1992. *Body and Emotion. The Aesthetics of Illness and Healing in the Nepal Himalayas*, Philadelphia, PA: University of Pennsylvania Press.

Devisch, R. 1991. 'Mediumistic divination among the Northern Yaka of Zaire'. In P. Peek (ed.) *African Divination Systems*. Bloomington, IN: Indiana University Press.

Dolgin, J. 2000. 'Choice, tradition and the new genetics: the fragmentation of the ideology of the family'. *Connecticut Law Review* 32: 523–66.

Donchin, A. and Purdy, L. (eds.) 1999. *Embodying Bioethics: Recent Feminist Advances*. Oxford: Rowman & Littlefield.

Doyle, R. 1997. *On Beyond Living: Rhetorical Transformations in the Life Sciences*. Stanford University Press.

Draper, E. 1991. *Risky Business: Genetic Testing and Exclusionary Practices in the Hazardous Workplace*. Cambridge University Press.

Duster, T. 1990. *Backdoor to Eugenics*. New York: Routledge.

Edel, M. and Edel, A. 1968 [1959]. *Anthropology and Ethics*, IL: Charles C. Thomas. 2nd edition.

Edelstein, L. 1967. 'Hippocratic prognosis'. In O. Temkin and C.L. Temkin (eds.) *Ancient Medicine: Selected Papers* by Ludwig Edelstein, pp. 65–110. Baltimore, MA: John Hopkins University Press.

Edwards, J. 2000. *Born and Bred: Idioms of Kinship and New Reproductive Technologies in England*. Oxford University Press.

Edwards, J., Franklin, S., Hirsch, E., Price, F., and Strathern, M. 1999. *Technologies of Procreation: Kinship in the Age of Assisted Conception*, 2nd edn., London: Routledge.

European Group on Ethics in Science and New Technologies to the European Commission 2003. *Opinion on the Ethical Aspects of Genetic Testing in the Workplace. (Opinion no. 18)* Luxembourg: Office for Official Publications of the European Communities.

European Society for Human Reproduction and Embryology 1999. 'ESHRE Preimplantation Genetic Diagnosis (PGD) Consortium: Preliminary Assessment of Data (1/97–9/98), *Human Reproduction* 14(12): 3138–48.

Evans Pritchard, E.E. 1967 [1937]. *Witchcraft, Oracles and Magic Among the Azande*. Oxford: Clarendon Press.

Evens, T.M.S. 1982. 'Two concepts of "society as a moral system": Evans-Pritchard heterodoxy', *Man* 17: 205–18.

Farmer, P. 1999. *Infections and Inequalities*, Berkeley, CA: University of California Press.

Farmer, P. 2003. *Pathologies of Power: Health, Human Rights, and the New War on the Poor*. Berkeley, CA: University of California Press.

Faubion, J. 2001. *The Ethics of Kinship: Ethnographic Inquiries*. Lanham, MD: Rowman & Littlefield Publishers.

Finkler, K. 2000. *Experiencing the New Genetics: Family and Kinship on the Medical Frontier*. Philadelphia, PA: University of Pennsylvania Press.

Finkler, K. 2003. 'Illusions of controlling the future: risk and genetic inheritance', *Anthropology and Medicine* 10(1): 59–70.

Firth, R. 1953. 'The study of values by social anthropologist', *Man* 231: 146–53.

Fluehr-Lobban, C. 2003. *Ethics and the Profession of Anthropology: Dialogue for a New Era*. Walnut Creek, CA: AltaMira Press, 2nd edn.

Foucault, M. 1966. 'Introduction' to G. Canguilhelm *Le Normal et la pathologique*. Paris: Presses Universitaires de France.

Foucault, M. 1970. *The Order of Things. An Archaeology of the Human Sciences*. London: Tavistock Publications.

Fox, R. 2000. 'Hearing where we're coming from – ethically and professionally'. In A.-M. Cantwell, Friedlander, E. and Tramm, M. (eds.) *Ethics and Anthropology. Facing Future Issues in Human Biology, Globalism, and Cultural Property*, pp. 1–8. New York: New York Academy of Sciences.

Fox, R.C. 1990. 'The evolution of American bioethics: a sociological perspective'. In G. Weisz (ed.) *Social Science Perspectives on Medical Ethics*, pp. 201–20. Dordrecht: Kluwer Academic Publishers.

Frank. G. 2000. *Venus on Wheels. Two Decades of Dialogue on Disability, Biography, and Being Female in America*, Berkeley, CA: University of California Press.

Frank, G., Blackhall, L.J., Michel, V., Murphy, S.T., Azen, S.P., and Park, K. 1998. 'A discourse of relationships in bioethics: patient autonomy and end-of-life decision-making among elderly Korean Americans', *Medical Anthropology Quarterly* 12(4): 403–23.

Frankenberg, R. 1980. 'Medical anthropology and development: a theoretical perspective', *Social Science and Medicine* 14B: 197–207.

Frankenberg, R. 1992. ' "Your time or mine": temporal contradictions of biomedical practice'. In R. Frankenberg (ed.) *Time, Health and Medicine*, pp. 1–30. London: Sage.

Frankenberg, R. and Leeson, J. 1976. 'Disease, illness and sickness: social aspects of the choice of healer in a Lusaka suburb'. In J.B. Loudon (ed.) *Social Anthropology and Medicine*, pp. 223–58. London: Academic Press.

Franklin, S. 1997. *Embodied Progress: A Cultural Account of Assisted Reproduction*, London: Routledge.

Franklin, S. and Lock. M. (eds.) 2003. *Remaking Life and Death: Toward an Anthropology of the Biosciences*. Sante Fe, NM: School of American Research Press.

Franklin, S. and Ragoné, H. (eds.) 1998. *Reproducing Reproduction: Kinship, Power and Technological Innovation*, Philadelphia, PA: University of Pennsylvania Press.

Fujimura, Joan H. 1996. *Crafting Science. A Sociohistory of the Quest for the Genetics of Cancer*. Cambridge, MA: Harvard University Press.

Galison, P. and D.J. Stump (eds.) 1996. *The Disunity of Science: Boundaries, Contexts and Power*. Stanford University Press.

Genetic Interest Group (1998). *Confidentiality Guidelines*, GIG: London.

GeneWatch UK 2002a. *Human Health and Genetics*. Parliamentary Briefing No.2 [April].

GeneWatch UK 2002b. ' "Genovations" genetic test kits'. Available at: http://www.genewatch.org/HumanGen/Tests/Tests_Intro.htm

GeneWatch UK 2003. *Genetic Testing in the Workplace*. A Report for GeneWatch UK by Kristina Staley, Buxton, Derbyshire: GeneWatch UK.

Gilham, I. and T. Rowland 2001. 'Predictive medicine: potential benefits from the integration of diagnostics and pharmaceuticals'. *International Journal of Medical Marketing* 2: 18–22.

Gillespie, S.D. 2000. 'Maya nested houses'. In R.A. Joyce and Gillespie S.D. (eds.) *Beyond Kinship: Social and Material Reproduction in House Societies*, pp. 135–60. University of Pennsylvania Press.

Gillon, R. (ed.) 1994. *Principles of Health Care Ethics*. New York: John Wiley & Sons.

Goffman, E. 1963. *Stigma*. New York: Simon and Schuster.

Good, Byron J. 1994. *Medicine, Rationality and Experience: An Anthropological Perspective*. Cambridge University Press.

Good, M.-J. Delvecchio, Brodwin, P.E., Good, B.J., and Kleinman A. (eds.) 1992. *Pain as Human Experience: An Anthropological Perspective*, Berkeley: University of California Press.

Goodman, A.H., Heath, D., and Lindee, S.M. (eds.) 2003. *Genetic Nature/Culture: Anthropology and Science Beyond the Two-Culture Divide*. Berkeley: University of California Press.

Gordon, D. 1990. 'Embodying illness, embodying cancer', *Culture, Medicine and Psychiatry* 14: 275–97.

Gordon, D. 1994. 'The ethics of ambiguity and concealment around cancer: interpretation of a local Italian world'. In P. Benner (ed.) *Interpretive Phenomenology: Embodiment, Caring and Ethics in Health and Illness*, Thousand Oaks, CA: Sage.

Gould, S.J. 2001. *Rocks of Ages. Science and Religion in the Fullness of Life*, London: Jonathan Cape.

Gray, A. 1995. *Genes and Generations: Living with Huntington's Disease*. Wellington: Huntington's Disease Association.

Green, J. 1995. 'Obstetricians' views on prenatal diagnosis and termination of pregnancy: 1980 compared with 1993', *British Journal of Obstetrics and Gynaecology* 102: 228–32.

Green, J.M., Richards, M., Murton, F., Statham, H., and Hallowell, N. 1997. 'Family communication and genetic counselling: the case of hereditary breast cancer and ovarian cancer', *Journal of Genetic Counselling* 6(1): 45–60.

Hacking, I. 1990. *The Taming of Chance*. Cambridge University Press.

Hahn, Robert A. 1995. *Sickness and Healing: An Anthropological Perspective*, London: Yale University Press.

Hahn, Robert A. and Atwood G. (eds.) 1985. *Physicians of Western Medicine. Anthropological Approaches to Theory and Practice*. Holland: D. Reidel.

Hamilton, W.D. 1964. 'The genetical evolution of social behaviour. I and II', *Journal of Theoretical Biology* 7: 1–16; 17–32.

Hamilton, W.D. 1975. 'Innate social aptitudes of man: an approach from evolutionary genetics'. In R. Fox (ed.) *Biosocial Anthropology*, pp. 133–57. New York: John Wiley Sons.

Haraway, D. 2000. *How Like A Leaf*. An Interview with Thyrza Nichols Goodeve. New York: Routledge.

Harper, P.S. 1996. *Huntington's Disease*. London: Saunders.

Harper, P.S. and Clarke, A. 1990. 'Should we test children for 'adult' genetic diseases?' *The Lancet* 335: 1205–6.

Harper, J.C. and Delhanty, J.D.A. 2000. 'Pre-Implantation genetic diagnosis', *Current Opinion in Obstetrics and Gynecology* 12: 67–72.

Harris, G. 1978. *Casting Out Anger: Religion Among the Taita of Kenya*. Cambridge University Press.

Hastrup, K. and Elsass, P. 1990. 'Anthropological advocacy. A contradiction in terms?', *Current Anthropology* 31(3): 301–11.

Hawkes, N. 2003. 'DIY healthcare – Britain's new £55 million hobby'. *The Times* 29 October, p. 3.

Hayden, M.R. 1981. *Huntington's Chorea*. Berlin: Springer-Verlag.

Hepburn, L. 1998. 'Genetic counselling: parental autonomy or acceptance of limits?' In M. Junker-kenny and L.S. Cahill (eds.) *The Ethics of Genetic Engineering*. London: SCM Press and Maryknoll, NY: Orbis Books.

Heyd, D. 1994. *Genethics. Moral Issues in the Creation of People*, Berkeley: University of California Press.

Higgs, R. 1998. 'Truth-telling'. In H. Kuhse and P. Singer (eds.) *A Companion to Bioethics*, pp. 432–40. Oxford: Blackwell.

Hodson, A. 1994. *Essential Genetics*. London: Bloomsbury.

Hoffmaster, B. 1990. 'Morality and the social sciences'. In G. Weisz (ed.) *Social Science Perspectives on Medical Ethics*, pp. 241–60. Dordrecht: Kluwer Academic Publishers.

Holtzman, N.A. and Marteau, T. 2000. 'Will genetics revolutionise medicine?', *New England Journal of Medicine* 343(2): 141–4 [13 July].

House of Commons Science and Technology Committee (1995). *Human Genetics: The Science and its Consequences* [Third Report]. London: HMSO.

House of Lords Select Committee on Science and Technology 2001. *Human Genetic Databases: Challenges and Opportunities*, 20 March, [4th Report]. London: HMSO.

Howell, S. 1997. 'Introduction'. In S. Howell (ed.). *The Ethnography of Moralities*, pp. 1–22. London: Routledge.

Howell, S. (ed.). *The Ethnography of Moralities*, London: Routledge.

Human Fertilisation and Embryology Authority and Advisory Committee on Genetic Testing 1999. *Consultation Document on Preimplantation Genetic Diagnosis*, HFEA/ACGT: London.

Human Fertilisation and Embryology Authority 2003. *Sex Selection: Options for Regulation*. London: HFEA.

Human Genetics Commission 2000. *Whose Hands on Your Genes? A Discussion Document on the Storage Protection and Use of Personal Genetic Information*, London: HGC.

Human Genetics Commission 2001. *Public Attitudes to Human Genetic Information*. People's Panel Quantitative Study conducted for the Human Genetics Commission. London: HGC.

Human Genetics Commission 2002. *Inside Information. Balancing Interests in the Use of Personal Genetic Data*. London: Department of Health.

Human Genetics Commission 2003. *Genes Direct. Ensuring the Effective Oversight of Genetic Tests Supplied Directly to the Public*. London: Department of Health.

Humphrey, C. 1997. 'Exemplars and rules: aspects of the discourse of moralities in Mongolia'. In S. Howell (ed.) *The Ethnography of Moralities*, pp. 25–47. London: Routledge.

Huntington's Disease Collaborative Research Group 1993. 'A novel gene containing a trinucleotide repeat that is expanded and unstable on Huntington's disease chromosome'. *Cell* 72: 971–83.

International Human Genome Mapping Consortium 2001. 'A physical map of the human genome', *Nature* 409: 934–41, (spec. issue on the human genome).

Jacobson-Widding, A. 1997. ' "I lied, I farted, I stole . . . .": dignity and morality in African discoures on personhood'. In S. Howell (ed.) *The Ethnography of Moralities*, pp. 48–73. London: Routledge.

Jackson, J.E. 2000. *Camp Pain: Talking with Chronic Pain Patients*, Philadelphia: University of Pennsylvania Press.

Jackson, J. 2001. *Truth, Trust and Medicine*, London: Routledge.

Jackson, M. 1982. *Allegories of the Wilderness: Ethics and Ambiguity in Kuranko Narratives*, Bloomington: Indiana University Press.

Jakobsen, M.D. 1999. *Shamanism: Traditional and Contemporary Approaches to the Masters of Spirits and Healing*. Oxford: Berghahn.

James, W. 1988. *The Listening Ebony: Moral Knowledge, Religion, and Power Among the Uduk of Sudan*. Oxford University Press and Clarendon Press.

James, W. 2000. 'Placing the unborn: on the social recognition of new life', *Anthropology and Medicine* 7(2): 169–89.

Jonsen, A. 1991. 'American moralism and the origins of bioethics in the United States', *Journal of Medicine and Philosophy* 16: 113–30.

Jules-Rosette, B. 1978. 'The veil of objectivity: prophecy, divination and social inquiry', *American Anthropologist* 80(3): 549–70.

Kay, L.E. 1993. *The Molecular Vision of Life: Caltech, the Rockefeller Foundation and the Rise of New Biology*. Oxford University Press.

Kay, L.E. 1999. 'In the beginning was the word?'. In M. Biagioli (ed.) *The Science Studies Reader*, pp. 224–33. London: Routledge.

Kay, L.E. 2000. *Who Wrote the Book of Life? A History of the Genetic Code*. Stanford University Press.

Keller, E. Fox. 1983. *A Feeling for the Organism: The Life and Work of Barbara McClintock*, New York: W.H. Freeman.

Keller, E. Fox. 1992. *Secrets of Life, Secrets of Death: Essays on Language, Gender and Science*. New York: Routledge.

Keller, E. Fox. 1995. *Refiguring Life: Metaphors of Twentieth Century Biology*. New York: Columbia University Press.

Kerr, A. 2003. 'Governing genetics: reifying choice and progress'. *New Genetics and Society* 22(2): 111–26.

Kerr, A. and Shakespeare, T. 2002. *Genetic Politics: From Eugenics to Genome*. Cheltenham: New Clarion Press.

Kessler, S. (ed.) 1979. *Genetic Counselling: Psychological Dimensions*. New York: Academic Press.

Kitcher, P. 1985. *Vaulting Ambition: Sociobiology and the Quest for Human Nature*, Cambridge, MA: MIT Press.

Kitcher, P. 1996. *The Lives to Come: The Genetic Revolution and Human Possibilities*. Harmondsworth: Penguin.

Klein, J. 1982. *Woody Guthrie: A Life*. New York: Ballantine Books.

Kleinman, A. 1978. 'Concepts and a model for the comparison of medical systems as cultural systems', *Social Science and Medicine B* 12: 85–93.

Kleinman, A. 1988. *The Illness Narratives: Suffering, Healing and the Human Condition*, New York: Basic Books.

Kleinman, A. 1995. *Writing at the Margin: Discourse Between Anthropology and Medicine*, Berkeley: University of California Press.

Kluckhohn, F. and Strodtbeck, F. 1961. *Variations in Value Orientations*. Evanston, IL: Row, Peterson.

Knorr-Cetina, K. 1999. *Epistemic Cultures: How the Sciences Make Knowledge*. Cambridge, MA: Harvard University Press.

Konrad, M. 2002. 'Pre-symptomatic networks: tracking experts across medical science and the new genetics'. In C. Shore and S. Nugent (eds.) *Elite Cultures: Anthropological Perspectives*, pp. 227–48. London: Routledge.

Konrad, M. 2003a. 'From secrets of life to the life of secrets: tracing genetic knowledge as genealogical ethics'. *Journal of the Royal Anthropological Institute* 9(2): 339–58.

Konrad, M. 2003b. 'Gifts of life in absentia: regenerative fertility and the puzzle of the "missing genetrix" '. In J. Haynes and J. Miller (eds.) *Inconceivable Conceptions: Psychotherapy, Fertility and the New Reproductive Technologies*, pp. 120–42. London: Routledge.

Konrad, M. 2003c. 'Predictive genetic testing and the making of the pre-symptomatic person: prognostic moralities amongst Huntington's affected families'. *Anthropology and Medicine* 10(1): 23–49.

Konrad, M. 2004. 'Offspring, being and wellbeing: parental decision making'. Paper presented to the Seminar on 'Human Reproduction. Selecting for Life: Scientific Basis and Policy Implications', Cambridge University Government Policy Programme, convened by Sir Gabriel Horn 23 April.

Konrad, M. (2005). *Nameless Relations: Anonymity, Melanesia and Reproductive Gift Exchange between British Ova Donors and Recipients*. Oxford: Berghahn.

Kuczewski, M. and Polansky, R. (eds.) 2000. *Bioethics. Ancient Themes in Contemporary Issues*. Cambridge, MA. MIT Press.

Kyle, D. 1985. *The Dancing Men*. Glasgow: Fontana Collins.

Laidlaw, J. 2002. 'For an anthropology of ethics and freedom'. *Journal of the Royal Anthropological Institute* 8(2): 311–32.

Lane, P.A. 1994. 'Targeted vs. universal screening'. In K. Seastone Stern and J.G. Davis (eds.) *Newborn Screening for Sickle Cell Disease: Issues and Implications*, pp. 157–60. New York: Council of Regional Networks for Genetic Services, Cornell University Medical College.

Last, M. 1981. 'The importance of knowing about non-knowing', *Social Science and Medicine* 15B: 387–92.

Latour, B. 1993. *We Have Never Been Modern*. Translated by C. Porter, Harvester: Wheatsheaf.

Leach, E. 1978. 'The proper study of mankind', *New Society*, 12 October, pp. 91–3.

Leach, E. 1981. 'Biology and social science: wedding or rape?', *Nature* 291: 267–68 (Review of C.L. Lumsden and E.O. Wilson 1981 *Genes, Mind and Culture: The Coevolutionary Process*.)

Leal-Pock, C. 1998. *Faces of Huntington's*. Ontario: Essence Publishing.

Lévi-Strauss, C. 1963. 'The effectiveness of symbols'. In *Structural Anthropology*, pp. 186–205. Harmondsworth, Middlesex: Penguin Books.

Lévi-Strauss, C. 1987. *Anthropology and Myth: Lectures 1951–1982*. Translated by R. Willis, Oxford: Blackwell.

Levitt, M. 1999. 'The ethics and impact on behaviour of knowledge about one's genome'. *British Medical Journal* 319: 1283.

Lewis, G. 1995. 'Revealed by illness: Aspects of the Gnau people's world and their perception of it'. In D. de Coppet and A. Iteanu (eds.) *Cosmos and Society in Oceania*, pp. 165–88. Oxford: Berghahn.

Lewis, G. 2000. *The Failure of Treatment*. Oxford University Press.

Lewontin, R.C., Rose, S., and Kamin, L. 1984. *Not in Our Genes*, New York: Pantheon Books.

Lewontin, R.C. 2000. *It Ain't Necessarily So: The Dream of the Human Genome and Other Illusions*. London: Granta Books.

Lieban, R.W. 1990. 'Medical anthropology and the comparative study of medical ethics'. In G. Weisz (ed.) *Social Science Perspectives on Medical Ethics*, pp. 221–40. Dordrecht: Kluwer Academic Publishers.

Lienhardt, G. 1969. *Divinity and Experience: The Religion of the Dinka*. Oxford: Clarendon Press.

Lippman, A. 1992. 'Led (astray) by genetic maps: the cartography of the human genome and health care'. *Social Science and Medicine* 35: 1469–76.

Lippman, A. 1993. 'Prenatal genetic testing and geneticization: Mother matters for all', *Fetal Diagnosis and Therapy* 8 (supp. 1): 175–88.

Lloyd, G.E.R. (ed.) 1978. 'Prognosis'. In *Hippocratic Writings*, trans. J. Chadwick and W.N. Mann, pp. 170–85. New York: Penguin.

Loch, L. 1999. 'Predictive genetic medicine – a new concept of disease'. In E. Hildt and S. Graumann (eds.) *Genetics in Human Reproduction*, pp. 185–96. Aldershot: Ashgate Publishing Ltd.

Lock, M. 1995. 'Contesting the natural in Japan: moral dilemmas and technologies of dying', *Culture, Medicine and Psychiatry* 19: 1–38.

Lock, M. 1998. 'Breast cancer. Reading the omens', *Anthropology Today* 14(4): 7–16.

Lock, M. and Gordon, D. (eds.) 1988. *Biomedicine Examined*. Dordrecht: Kluwer Academic Publishers.

Lock, M. and Kaufert, P.A. (eds.) 1998. *Pragmatic Women and Body Politics*. Cambridge University Press.

Macintyre, B. 2003. 'Labour's hypocritical oath: patient, heal thyself', *The Times*. 4 June 2003, p. 2.

Malinowksi, B. 1978 [1935]. *Coral Gardens and Their Magic*, (volume II), New York: Dover Publications.

Mange, E.J. and Mange, A.P. 1999. *Basic Human Genetics*, MA: Sinauer Associates.

Marshall, P. and Koenig, B. 1996. 'Bioethics in anthropology: perspectives on culture, medicine and morality'. In C. Sargent and T.M. Johnson (eds.) *Medical Anthropology. Contemporary Theory and Method*, pp. 349–73. New York: Greenwood Press.

Marshall, P., Thomasma, D, and O'Keefe, P. 1991. 'Disclosing HIV status: ethical issues explored', *Journal of the American Dental Association* 122: 11–15.

Marteau, T. and Richards, M. (eds.) 1996. *The Troubled Helix. Social and Psychological Implications of the New Human Genetics*. Cambridge University Press.

Mathew, C. 2001. 'Postgenomic technologies: hunting the genes for common disorders'. *BMJ* 322: 1031–34 [28 April].

Mattingly, C. 1998. *Healing Dramas and Clinical Plots: The Narrative Structure of Experience*. Cambridge University Press.

Mauss, M. 1990 [1925]. *The Gift. The Form and Reason for Exchange in Archaic Societies*, trans. W.D. Halls, London: Routledge.

McCallum, C. 1996. 'The body that knows: from Cashinahua epistemology to a medical anthropology of lowland South America', *Medical Anthropology Quarterly* 10(3): 347–72.

McCallum, C. 2001. *Gender and Sociality in Amazonia: How Real People Are Made*. Oxford: Berghahn.

Medick, H. and Sabean, D. (eds.) 1984. *Interest and Emotion: Essays on the Study of Family and Kinship*. Cambridge University Press.

Meissen, G.J. and Berchek, R.L. 1987. Intended use of predictive testing by those at risk of HD, *American Journal of Medical Genetics* 26: 283–93.

Melzer, D. and Zimmern, R. 2002. 'Genetics and medicalisation'. *British Medical Journal* 324: 863–4.

Michie, S. and Marteau, T. 1996. 'Genetic counselling: some issues of theory and practice'. In T. Marteau and M. Richards (eds.) *The Troubled Helix: Social and Psychological Implications of the New Human Genetics*, pp. 104–22. Cambridge University Press.

Middleton, J. 1971. 'Oracles and divination among the Lugbara'. In M. Douglas and P. Kaberry (eds.) *Man in Africa*, pp. 161–78. New York: Doubleday Anchor.

Mol, A.M. and Berg, M. 1998. 'Differences in medicine: an introduction'. In M. Berg and A. Mol (eds.) *Differences in Medicine. Unravelling Practices, Techniques, and Bodies*, Durham and London: Duke University Press.

Monks, J. 2000. 'Talk as social suffering: narratives of talk in medical settings', *Anthropology & Medicine* 7(1): 15–38.

Morgan, W. 1931. 'Navaho treatment of sickness: diagnosticians', *American Anthropologist* (33): 390–402.

Moynihan, R., Heath, I., and Henry, D. 2002. 'Selling sickness: the pharmaceutical industry and disease mongering'. *British Medical Journal* 324: 886–91.

Muller, J. 1994. 'Anthropology, bioethics, and medicine: a provocative trilogy', *Medical Anthropology Quarterly* 8(4): 448–67.

Murray, T.H. 1997. 'Genetic exceptionalism and "future diaries": is genetic information different from other medical information?'. In M.A. Rothstein (ed.) *Genetic Secrets: Protecting Privacy and Confidentiality in the Genetic Era*, pp. 60–73. New Haven and London: Yale University Press.

Nader, L. (ed.) 1996. *Naked Science: Anthropological Inquiry into Boundaries, Power and Knowledge*. London: Routledge.

Nelkin, D. 1996. 'The science wars: responses to a marriage failed', *Social Text 46/47*, 14 (1–2): 93–100.

Nelkin, D. and Tancredi, L. 1989. *Dangerous Diagnostics: The Social Power of Biological Information*. New York: Basic Books.

Nelson, H. Lindemann. 1997. *Stories and Their Limits: Narrative Approaches to Bioethics*. New York: Routledge.

Nietzsche, F. 1873. 'On truth and lying in an extra-moral sense'. In S.L. Gilman, C. Blair, and D.J. Parent (eds.) 1989. *Friedrich Nietzsche on Rhetoric and Language*, pp. 246–57. Oxford University Press.

Noddings, N. 1984. *Caring: A Feminine Approach to Ethics and Moral Education*, Berkeley: University of California Press.

Novas, C. and Rose, N. 2000. 'Genetic risk and the birth of the somatic individual'. *Economy and Society* 29(4): 485–513.

Nowotny, H., Scott, P., and Gibbons, M. 2002. *Re-thinking Science: Knowledge and the Public in an Age of Uncertainty*. Cambridge: Polity Press.

Nuffield Council on Bioethics 1998. *Mental Disorders and Genetics: The Ethical Context*. London: NCB.

Nuffield Council on Bioethics 1993. *Genetic Screening: Ethical Issues*. London: NCB.

Nuffield Council on Bioethics 2002. *Genetics and Human Behaviour: The Ethical Context*. London: NCB.

Nukaga, Y. 2002. 'Between tradition and innovation in new genetics: the continuity of medical pedigrees and the development of combination work in the case of Huntington's disease'. *New Genetics and Society* 21(1): 39–64.

Nyberg, D. 1993. *The Varnished Truth: Truth Telling and Deceiving in Ordinary Life*. University of Chicago Press.

Okely, J. and H. Callaway (eds.) 1992. *Anthropology and Autobiography*, London: Routledge.

Olby, R. 1974. *The Path to the Double Helix*. London: Macmillan.

Overing, J. and Passes, A. (eds.) 2000. *The Anthropology of Love and Anger: The Aesthetics of Conviviality in Native Amazonia*. London: Routledge.

Park, G.K. 1963. 'Divination and its social contexts', *Journal Royal Anthropological Institute* 93: 195–209.

Parkin, D. 1985. 'Introduction'. In D. Parkin (ed.) *The Anthropology of Evil*, Oxford: Basil Blackwell.

Parsons, E.P. and Atkinson, P.A. 1992. 'Lay constructions of genetic risk'. *Sociology of Health and Illness* 14: 437–55.

Pauling, L. 1968. 'Reflections on the new biology', *UCLA Law Review* (15): 267–72.

Peek, P. (ed.) 1991. *African Divination Systems*. Bloomington, IL: Indiana University Press.

Pellegrino, E. 1992. 'Intersections of western biomedical ethics and world culture'. In E. Pellegrino, P. Mazzarella, and P. Corsi (eds.) *Transcultural Dimensions in Medical Ethics*, Frederick, MD: University Publishing Group.

Pelias, M. 1991. 'Duty to disclose in medical genetics: a legal perspective', *American Journal of Human Genetics* 39: 347–54.

Petersen, A. and Bunton, R. 2002. *The New Genetics and the Public's Health*. London: Routledge.

Pocock, D. 1986. 'The ethnography of morals', *International Journal of Moral and Social Studies* 1(1): 3–20.

Popper, K. 1959. *The Logic of Scientific Discovery*, New York: Basic Books.

Press, N.A. and Browner, C.H. 1994. 'Collective silences, collective fictions: how prenatal diagnostic testing became part of routine prenatal care'. In K.H. Rothenberg and E.J. Thomson (eds.) *Women and Prenatal Testing: Facing the Challenges of Genetic Technology*, Columbus, OH: Ohio State University Press.

Proctor, R. 1992. 'Genomics and eugenics: how fair is the comparison?' In G.J. Annas and S. Elias (eds.) *Gene Mapping: Using Law and Ethics as Guides*, pp. 57–93. New York: Oxford University Press.

Quarell, O.W., Tyler, A., Upadhyaya, M., Meredith, A.L., Youngman, S., and Harper, P.S. 1987. 'Exclusion testing for Huntington's Disease in pregnancy with a closely linked DNA marker', *The Lancet*, (i), 1281–3.

Rabinow, P. 1992. 'Artificiality and enlightenment: from sociobiology to biosociality'. In J. Crary and S. Kwinter (eds.) *Incorporations*, pp. 234–52. New York: Zone.

Rabinow, P. 1996. *Making PCR: A Story of Biotechnology*. University of Chicago Press.

Rabinow, P. 1999. *French DNA. Trouble in Purgatory*. University of Chicago Press.

Rapp, R. 1989. 'Chromosomes and communication: the discourse of genetic counselling'. In L.M. Whiteford and M.L. Poland (eds.) *New Approaches to Human Reproduction*, pp. 25–41, Boulder, CO: Westview Press.

Rapp, R. 1991. 'Moral pioneers: women, men and fetuses on the frontier of reproductive technology'. In M. di Leonardo (ed.) *Gender at the Crossroads of Knowledge: Feminist Anthropology in the Postmodern Era*, pp. 383–95. Berkeley: University of California Press.

Rapp, R. 1995. 'Heredity, or: revising the facts of life'. In C. Delaney and S. Yanagisako (eds.) *Naturalising Power*, pp. 69–86. London: Routledge.

Rapp, R. 1997. 'Real-time fetus'. In G. Lee Downey and J. Dumit (eds.) *Cyborgs and Citadels: Anthropological Interventions in Emerging Sciences and Technologies*, pp. 31–48. Santa Fe, NM: School of American Research Press.

Rapp, R. 1999. *Testing Women, Testing the Fetus: The Social Impact of Amniocentesis in America*. New York: Routledge.

Read, K. 1955. 'Morality and the concept of the person among the Gahuku-Gama', *Oceania*, xxv (4): 233–82.

Reed-Danahay, D.E. (ed.) 1997. *Auto/Ethnography: Rewriting the Self and the Social*, Oxford: Berghahn.

Richards, M. 1997. 'It runs in the family: lay knowledge about inheritance'. In A. Clarke and E. Parsons (eds.) *Culture, Kinship and Genes*, pp. 175–94. London: Macmillan Press.

Rifkin, J. 1998. *The Biotech Century: How Genetic Commerce Will Change the World*. London: Phoenix.

Rivers, W.H.R. [1910] 1968. 'The genealogical method of anthropological inquiry'. In *Kinship and Social Organisation*, L.S.E. Monographs in Social Anthropology, 34: 97–109. London: The Athlone Press.

Rivers, W.H.R. [1914] 1968. 'Classificatory terminology and cross-cousin marriage'. In *Kinship and Social Organisation*, L.S.E. Monographs in Social Anthropology, 34: 39–54. London: The Athlone Press.

Rosaldo, M.Z. 1980. *Knowledge and Passion: Ilongot Conceptions of Self and Social Life*, New York: Cambridge University Press.

Rose, H. and Rose, S. (eds.) 2000. *Alas, Poor Darwin: Arguments Against Evolutionary Psychology*. New York: Harmony Books.

Rose, N. 1990. *Governing the Soul. The Shaping of the Private Self.* London: Routledge.

Rose, N. 1999. *Powers of Freedom: Reframing Political Thought.* Cambridge University Press.

Rose, S. 1997. *Lifelines: Biology, Freedom, Determinism.* Harmondsworth: Penguin Books.

Rothman, B.K. 1986. *The Tentative Pregnancy: Prenatal Diagnosis and the Future of Motherhood.* New York: Viking Press.

Rothman, B.K. 1998. *Genetic Maps and Human Imaginations: The Limits of Science in Understanding Who We Are.* New York: Norton.

Rothman, D. 1991. *Strangers at the Bedside: a History of How Law and Bioethics Transformed Medical Decision-Making*, New York: Basic Books.

Rothstein, M. (ed.) *Genetic Secrets. Protecting Privacy and Confidentiality in the Genetic Era.* New Haven: Yale University Press.

Rubalcaba, J. 1996. *Saint Vitus Dance.* New York: Clarion Books.

Sawyer, R. 1998. *Frameshift.* New York: Tor Books.

Scheper-Hughes, N. 1995. 'The primacy of the ethical', *Current Anthropology* 36(3): 409–20.

Schulman, J., Black, S., Handyside, A.H., and Nance, W. 1996. 'Preimplantation genetic testing for Huntington's disease and certain other dominantly inherited disorders', *Clinical Genetics* 49: 57–8.

Segerstråle, Ullica. 2001. *Defenders of the Truth. The Sociobiology Debate.* Oxford University Press.

Sermon. K., Goossens, V., Seneca, S., Lissens, W., de Vos, A., Vandervorst, M., van Steirteghern, A., and Liebaers, I. 1998. 'Preimplantation diagnosis for Huntington's Disease: clinical application and analysis of the HD expansion in affected embryos', *Prenatal Diagnosis* (18): 1427–36.

Shakespeare, T. 1999. 'Losing the plot: medical and activist discourses of the contemporary genetics of disability'. In P. Conrad and J. Gabe (eds.) *Sociological Perspectives on the New Genetics*, pp. 171–90. Oxford: Blackwell.

Shakespeare, T. 1998. 'Choices and rights: eugenics, genetics and disability equality'. *Disability and Society* 13(5): 665–81.

Shaw, R. 1991. 'Splitting truths from darkness: espistemological aspects of Temne divination' In P. Peek (ed.) *African Divination Systems*. Bloomington, IN: Indiana University Press.

Shore, B. 1990. 'Human ambivalence and the structuring of human values', *Ethos* 18(12): 165–79.

Singer, M. 1992. 'The application of theory in medical anthropology: an introduction', *Medical Anthropology* 14: 1–8.

Silvers, A. 1999. 'On not iterating women's disability: a crossover perspective on genetic dilemmas'. In A. Donchin and L.M. Purdy (eds.) *Embodying Bioethics: Recent Feminist Advances*, pp. 177–202. Lanham, MD: Rowman & Littlefield Publishers.

Sinsheimer, R. 1976. *The Book of Life*. Reading, MA: Addison-Wesley.

Skultans, V. (ed.) 2000. 'Narrative illness and the body', *Anthropology and Medicine*, 7(1) [special issue].

Slomka, J. 1992. 'The negotiation of death: clinical decision-making at the end of life', *Social Science and Medicine* 35(3): 251–9.

Strathern, M. 1968. 'Popokl: the question of morality', *Mankind* 6(11): 553–62.

Strathern, M. 1991. *Partial Connections*. Lanham, MD: Rowman and Littlefield Publishers.

Strathern, M. 1992a. *Reproducing the Future: Essays on Anthropology, Kinship and the New Reproductive Technologies*. Manchester University Press.

Strathern, M. 1992b. *After Nature*. Cambridge University Press.

Strathern, M. 1995. 'Nostalgia and the new genetics'. In D. Battaglia (ed.) *Rhetorics of Self-Making*, pp. 97–120. Berkeley, CA: University of California Press.

Strathern, M. (ed.) 2000. *Audit Cultures: Anthropological Studies in Accountability, Ethics and the Academy*. London: Routledge.

Sudbery, P. 1998. *Human Molecular Genetics*, Harlow: Longman.

Suter, S.M. 1993. 'Whose genes are these anyway? Familial conflicts over access to genetic information', *Michigan Law Review*: 1854–908.

Suzuki, D. and Knudtson, P. 1990. *Genethics: The Clash Between The New Genetics And Human Values*, Cambridge, MA: Harvard University Press.

Taussig, M. 1987. *Shamanism, Colonialism and the Wild Man*. University of Chicago Press.

Taussig, M. 1980. 'Reification and the consciousness of the patient', *Social Science and Medicine* B:14: 3–13.

Tibbens, A., Niermeijer, M.F., and Roos, R.A.C., 1992. 'Understanding the low uptake of presymptomatic DNA testing for Huntington's disease', *The Lancet* 340: 1416.

Tokar, B. (ed.) 2001. *Redesigning Life? The Worldwide Challenge to Genetic Engineering*, London: Zed Books.

Tolmie, J.L., Davidson, H.R., May, H.M., McIntosh, K., Paterson, J.S., and Smith, B. 1995. 'The prenatal exclusion test for Huntington's Disease: experience in the west of Scotland, 1986–1993', *Journal of Medical Genetics* 32: 97–101.

Tong, R. 1997. *Feminist Approaches to Bioethics. Theoretical Reflections and Practical Applications*. Boulder, CO: Westview Press.

Traweek, S. 1992. 'Border crossings: narratives strategies in science studies and among physicists in Tsukuba science city, Japan'. In A. Pickering (ed.) *Science as Practice and Culture*. University of Chicago, 429–66.

Tröhler, U. and Reiter-Theil, S. (eds.) 1998. *Ethics Codes in Medicine: Foundations and Achievements of Codification since 1947*. Aldershot: Ashgate Publishing Ltd.

Turner, V. 1975. *Revelation and Divination in Ndembu Ritual*. Ithaca, NY: Cornell University Press.

Tyler, A., Quarrell, O., Lazarou, L., Meredith, A., and Harper, P. 1990. 'Exclusion testing in pregnancy for Huntington's Disease', *Journal of Medical Genetics* (27): 488–95.

UNESCO 1997a. *Universal Declaration on the Human Genome and Human Rights*, Paris: UNESCO.

UNESCO 1997b. *Final Report* of the Committee of Governmental Experts for the Finalisation of a Declaration on the Human Genome, 22–25 July, Paris.

Utley, A. 2003. 'Spot the university candidate – aged 3'. *The Times Higher Education Supplement*. September 19, pp. 1–2.

Venter, C., Adams, D., Myerss, W., Li, W., Mural, J., and Sutton, G. 2001. 'The sequence of the human genome', *Science* 291: 1304–51.

Venter, C. *et al.* 2001. *Science*, 291: 1304–51, (spec. issue on the human genome).

Vine, B. 1989. *The House of Stairs*. New York: Harmony Books.

Visweswaran, K. 1994. *Fictions of Feminist Ethnography*, Minneapolis, MN: University of Minnesota Press.

Vitebsky, P. 1995. *The Shaman*. London: Little, Brown.

Watson, J. 1980. *The Double Helix*. New York: W.W. Norton.

Werbner, R.P. 1989. 'Tswapong wisdom divination: making the hidden seen'. In *Ritual Passage, Sacred Journey: The Process and Organisation of Religious Movement*. Washington, DC: Smithsonian Institution Press.

Wexler, A. 1996. *Mapping Fate: A Memoir of Family, Risk, and Genetic Research*. Berkeley, CA: University of California Press.

Wexler, N. Sabin 1979. 'Genetic Russian roulette: the experience of being at risk for Huntington's disease'. In S. Kessler (ed.) *Genetic Counselling: Psychological Dimensions*. New York: Academic Press.

Wexler, N. Sabin 1989. 'The oracle of DNA'. In L.P. Rowland (ed.) *Molecular Genetics of Neuromuscular Disease*. Oxford University Press.

Wexler, N. Sabin 1992. 'Clairvoyance and caution: repercussions from the Human Genome Project'. In D.J. Kevles and L. Hood (eds.) *The Code of Codes*, pp. 211–43. Cambridge, MA.: Harvard University Press.

Whyte, S. Reynolds 1991. 'Power and knowledge in Nyole divination'. In P. Peek (ed.) *African Divination Systems*. Bloomington, IN: Indiana University Press.

Whyte, S. Reynolds 1997. *Questioning Misfortune. The Pragmatics of Uncertainty in Eastern Uganda*. Cambridge University Press.

Wiggins S., Whyte, P. *et al.* 1992. 'The psychological consequences of predictive testing for Huntington's Disease', *New England Journal of Medicine* 327/20: 1401–5.

Wilson, E. 1975. *Sociobiology: The New Synthesis*. Cambridge, MA: Belknap Press of Harvard University Press.

Wilson, E. 1978. *On Human Nature*. Cambridge, MA: Harvard University Press.

Wilson, E.O. 1998. *Consilience: The Unity of Knowledge*. London: Little, Brown.

Wolf, S. (ed.) 1996. *Feminism and Bioethics: Beyond Reproduction*. Oxford University Press.

World Health Organisation 2002. *Genomics and World Health. Report of the Advisory Committee on Health Research*. Geneva: WHO.

Yoder, P. S. 1997. 'Negotiating relevance: belief, knowledge, and practice in international health projects', *Medical Anthropology Quarterly* 11(2): 131–46.

Young, K. 1997. *Presence in the Flesh: The Body in Medicine*, Cambridge, MA: Harvard University Press.

Young, A. 1982. 'The Anthropologies of Illness and Sickness', *Annual Review of Anthropology* 11: 257–85.

Zimmerli, W.C. 1990. 'Who has the right to know the genetic constitution of a particular person?'. In R. Chadwick and G. Bock (eds.) *Human Genetic Information: Science, Law and Ethics*, pp. 93–102. Chichester: John Wiley & Sons.

Zola, I.K. 1972. 'Medicine as an institution of social control', *Sociological Review*, 20(4)[n.s.]: 487–509.

Index

Printed in the United States
by Baker & Taylor Publisher Services

Printed in the United States
by Baker & Taylor Publisher Services